Healing
Anxiety

Harmony ❧ Health ❧ Happiness

Healing Anxiety

A natural approach to managing
anxiety, worry, and fear

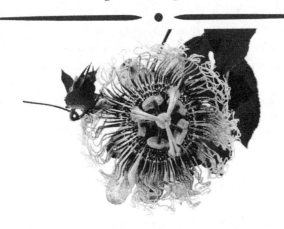

Dominga Nunez, ND, CNHP

Espaillat Publications
HealingBodiesandMinds.com

For bulk orders, contact espaillatpublications@gmail.com.

The information in this book is not intended to diagnose, treat, cure, or prevent any disease, nor should it replace the services of a licensed healthcare provider. Before using herbal products or starting any type of program, consult with a qualified healthcare practitioner or talk with your doctor, especially if you are pregnant, nursing, or on any medications, or if you are planning to administer herbal products to a child. This book is for educational purposes only; neither the author nor publisher is responsible for any adverse effect resulting from the use of its content.

ISBN: 978-1-7355816-0-6
ISBN: 978-1-7355816-1-3 (ebook)

This book is dedicated first to my Lord and Savior Jesus Christ. He has been my strength to keep me going and my refuge in times of despair.

I also dedicate this book to all those who are suffering from anxiety. My heart goes out to all of you.

To all the people in my life who believed in me and are always with me in the good and the bad. To Frank, my husband, for his support; Bryant and Kenneth, who make me proud; my two sisters, Agueda and Monica, and my niece, Greeny, who are my spiritual strength.

"Health is the greatest of human blessings."

~ Hippocrates

Contents

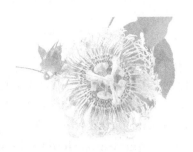

Chapter 1

My Journey

My first experience with debilitating anxiety occurred many years ago. I was a single working mother of two young boys living a normal life in London when I began experiencing several frightening symptoms including heart palpitations, shortness of breath, and insomnia. The symptoms seemed to come out of nowhere.

A doctor conducted a wide range of tests and concluded there was nothing physically wrong with me. Still, I was increasingly anxious and fearful. After several months, I decided to go to the United States where I saw several doctors, including a cardiologist, who told me the same thing: All the tests came back normal; my heart was healthy. I returned to London anxious, confused, and afraid. It was more than a year after my initial symptoms, and I had no answers and nowhere to turn for help.

Shortly after arriving home, I got very sick. My heart rate accelerated, my chest was tight, I was having a hard time breathing, my left arm was numb, and I felt a tingling up and down my legs. I called the paramedics. As they checked me out, they asked me a few questions, then told me I was having a panic attack.

That only increased my confusion. I was healthy and didn't have any unusual stress in my life. There was no reason for me to feel panicked and, besides, how can a panic attack do all that? I was sure it had to be something more serious, but what?

My symptoms subsided, and the paramedics left. After a while, the symptoms returned. I didn't want to call the paramedics again, but I was terrified. I was so afraid I was going to die that I wrote a letter to my kids so they would know what to do if they found me dead.

I made it through that awful night. The next day, I felt like I'd been given a second chance—and I realized it was going to be up to me to figure out what was going on. My search began with a book on natural remedies that I had bought a few years before. The book listed conditions alphabetically. It didn't take me long to reach the word *anxiety*. I only had to read a little further to realize that's what I had. With that understanding, it seemed possible that I would finally find some answers.

My research revealed that I was doing some of the things that can cause or exacerbate anxiety, including consuming too much caffeine and not getting enough sleep. I began making changes, saw immediate results, and, in just a few days, my symptoms disappeared.

While that may sound like a happy ending, it wasn't. There's more to my story.

Life went on. I moved to the United States and got married. Seventeen years after my first anxiety attack, I had another one. The condition was back with a vengeance, more intense than before and accompanied by new symptoms. I was afraid to be alone and yet afraid to leave the house. Other new symptoms included dizziness, dry mouth, shakiness, cold chills, and a feverish sensation, yet I didn't actually have a fever. Even though I knew it might be anxiety, I was confused by the additional symptoms and tried to push through it.

Then one day, while driving to work, I felt like I was losing control of everything. I didn't want to hold the steering wheel, my arms were weak, and I felt incapacitated. My heart was pounding and racing, my chest was tight, my mouth was dry, and my arms and legs were tingling. I was able to stop my car safely and call 911. When the paramedics arrived, they checked me out and told me my blood pressure was perfect and I was fine. I went home, thinking that a day of rest was all I needed.

I was wrong. Things only got worse. In addition to the physical symptoms, I became afraid of so many things—irrational fears that caused me to stop working for nearly two years. Nightmares kept me from sleeping, light and bright colors bothered me, I couldn't hold a conversation for longer than three minutes. I was easily tired and scared, I developed insomnia, and my muscles stayed tensed, which created intense muscle pain and constant dizziness. I was short of breath, I felt a lump in my throat, and my heart rate was constantly accelerated. The effects of anxiety consumed my life. Thank God for my husband, who not only stepped up to care for me but also everything else in our home while I searched for a solution.

Gradually, through prayer and alternative medicine, I

was able to heal and lead a normal life again. I continued my study of anxiety and developed a deeper understanding of the condition and the various remedies and therapies available, and I want to share what I have learned.

If you or someone you love suffers from anxiety, know that there is help, there are solutions, and we can conquer this debilitating condition.

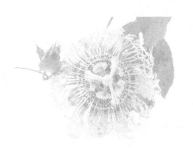

Chapter 2

What is Anxiety?

Anxiety is defined as *an apprehensive uneasiness or nervousness usually over an impending or anticipated ill: a state of being anxious.* According to the National Institute of Mental Health (NIMH), anxiety disorders are the most common mental illness in the United States, affecting 40 million adults age 18 and older, or 18 percent of the population. That's a lot of people!

When someone has experienced anxiety for an extended period or if it is severe enough, it can transform into panic attacks. The symptoms of a panic attack may include:

- a sudden feeling of panic and fear
- restlessness
- uneasiness
- cold or sweaty hands or feet
- numbness in the hands or feet

- tingling in arms or legs
- shortness of breath
- increased heart rate
- heart palpitations
- dizziness
- feeling faint
- chest tightness and/or pain
- dry mouth
- hot flashes or chills
- trembling
- insomnia
- nightmares
- muscle tension which can develop into muscle aches
- irritability
- sweating
- a fear of dying
- constant worry
- lump or choking feeling in throat

Even though these symptoms may sound far-fetched or crazy, they exist and are real. If you've never had an anxiety or panic attack, it's difficult, if not impossible, to understand what it feels like. The simple words describing the physical sensations don't come even close to the range of actual feelings that are experienced simultaneously when an anxiety attack is happening.

Anxiety can be debilitating. It takes control of your ability to perform everyday tasks, it robs you of quality of life, it negatively impacts your productivity on the job, it disrupts relationships, and ultimately deteriorates your health and life. It takes strength and determination to seize control of anxiety and manage it.

The symptoms of anxiety can manifest gradually

or suddenly, with or without warning. Some people will experience all the above symptoms at the same time; others will experience several but not all; still others will experience just a few.

It's essential to recognize the difference between merely feeling anxious and an actual anxiety attack. Anxious feelings are generally short-term and focused on something specific. For example, you may feel anxious if you have to make a speech or an important presentation at work. You may feel anxious while you wait for results from an exam, if you're starting a new job or new school, or if you're moving. Sometimes external events ranging from political issues to natural disasters can make us anxious. These are normal, common stressors that affect most people temporarily. Even though you're feeling agitated and unsettled, you understand why, and you are still in control of yourself.

"Failure isn't falling down. It's staying down."
      Mary Pickford

An anxiety attack has its own set of symptoms that can start abruptly without any apparent cause. Anxiety attacks are physically and emotionally devastating. Sufferers feel like they're losing control of their mental faculties and environment, and they don't know why. It's common to need emergency care at this point. Beyond the physical indicators listed above, anxiety often causes people to develop unexplained fears and even phobias, such as fear of large groups, fear of being confined in a small space like an elevator or public transportation, fear of leaving one's home, fear of water, heights, spiders, the dark—the list goes on. A person may suddenly become afraid of something he had routinely done without any problems before or may find that familiar daily routines have suddenly become complicated and frightening.

Approximately twelve different anxiety disorder sub-types are known by clinicians. The main ones are panic disorder, generalized anxiety, phobias, obsessive-compulsive disorder, and post-traumatic stress syndrome. Some of the more common symptoms of these disorders include:

Panic attack disorder symptoms: Rapid pounding heart rate, trembling and shaking, hot flashes and chills, shortness of breath, sweating, fear of losing control and dying, feeling of impending doom and danger, tightness on the chest, and a choking sensation.

Phobias: Similar to panic attack, including accelerated heart rate, trembling, choking sensation, chest tightness and pain, heart palpitations, dry mouth, dizziness, tingling in arms and legs, hot flashes and chills, rapid breathing, sweating.

Obsessive symptoms: Persistent and negative or intrusive thoughts, fear of hurting someone you love or images of hurting someone you love, thoughts of causing other harm, fear of germ contamination, persistent sexual thoughts and recurring unwanted thoughts, hypervigilance, panic of losing or not having things you might need.

Compulsive symptoms: Positioning objects to face in a specific way, continually checking things like stove knobs or door locks, frequently washing or cleaning hands or items, ritualistic conducts.

Post-traumatic stress syndrome: Severe anxiety, depression, unwanted memories of the trauma, nightmares, insomnia, anticipation of situations that might bring back memories of the trauma, guilt, loneliness, emotional detachment, irritability, hostility, social isolation and loss of interest for places and activities, self-destructive behavior.

Generalized anxiety disorder: Persistent worry, trouble concentrating, restlessness, fatigue, hyperventilating, irritability, unwanted thoughts, fear, anxiousness, heart palpitations, headaches, difficulty falling asleep, trembling, constant thoughts, muscle tension, and back pain.

How the nervous system responds to anxiety

When we experience stress or anxiety, we experience symptoms such as tensed muscles, heart rate acceleration,

PARASYMPATHETIC AND SYMPATHETIC NERVOUS SYSTEMS

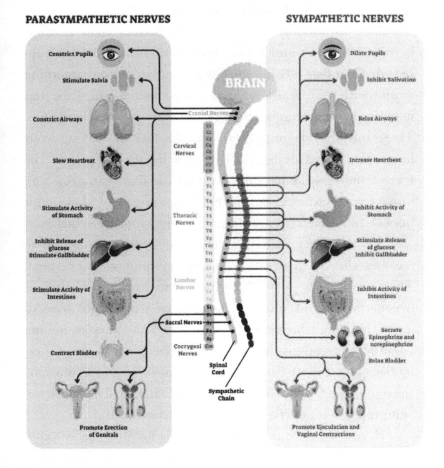

PARASYMPATHETIC NERVES   **SYMPATHETIC NERVES**

high blood pressure, etc. These symptoms are normal body responses to help the body deal with the stress, and this stress response comes from the sympathetic nervous system, which controls the body's responses to threats or danger. The parasympathetic nervous system keeps our bodies from overworking and restores us to a calm state. These two systems have opposite functions. For example, the sympathetic nervous system fires up our "fight or flight" response and prepares us for action. The parasympathetic nervous system helps us slow down, relax, and "rest and digest"; it controls functions of the body when it's resting.

After an anxiety attack, you can become more anxious because you don't understand how it started and why it happened. Then fear sets in—fear that there might be something wrong with you, fear that it might happen again, fear that negative things are going to happen to you or your loved ones. These initial fears might include the fear of leaving your home, the fear of dying, the fear of being around people, the fear of noises—the list goes on, and the fears can grow and impact your life and relationships. You might develop major insecurities driven by your fear of having another attack.

Some anxiety sufferers feel nervous all the time for no reason—they're just edgy, and everything startles them. They may have negative thoughts and nightmares. Their lives become a cycle of anguish, pessimism, worry, and fear—a cycle they can't break. Others may feel like they're having what is commonly called a nervous breakdown because their bodies can't cope with the intense emotions and symptoms they're feeling. The panic they go through daily causes the symptoms to intensify, creating a downward spiral.

If any of this sounds familiar, either because you've experienced it or you've seen it in someone you love, know that there is hope and help. It begins with understanding what has created an epidemic of anxiety. We are constantly on the go, we live a fast life where we don't have time to sit and enjoy healthy meals in a relaxed way, we work long hours, we depend on stimulants like caffeine to keep us awake and functioning, we sleep very little, and get up very early to repeat the pattern all over again. As the damage builds, this pattern can lead to a panic attack or an anxiety attack. Though it may seem like it came on suddenly, in reality, it was developing for months or even years. Sleep deprivation, excessive caffeine consumption, not eating a balanced diet with the right kind of nutrients—all this can deplete the brain and the body, and eventually affect the adrenal glands and nervous system.

To control and finally eliminate anxiety, we must first get to the source. In the next chapter, we'll examine what causes anxiety.

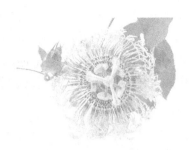

Chapter 3

What Causes Anxiety and Who Gets It?

While anxiety can be brought on by several factors, the number one cause is chronic stress.

Constant stress negatively affects the nervous system and the immune system. It can derail normal body functions and disrupt hormonal activity. Stress can also affect the production of mood-involving neurotransmitters like serotonin and dopamine. When the body is under stress, it increases the production of the stress hormone cortisol. Elevated cortisol levels reduce serotonin and dopamine, which are the two brain chemicals responsible for mood, sleep, energy, appetite, and sex drive. Serotonin makes us feel good and happy while dopamine stimulates us to get up, do things, and keep going. When these two neurotransmitters are low, we can experience anxiety, depression, lack of motivation, reduced enthusiasm, and feel tired and sluggish. Unresolved stress can result in insomnia, impaired sleep, and a wide range of other health complaints. Studies show that stress can raise serum lipids and lead to heart disease.Other causes of anxiety include:

- Hormonal imbalances
- Financial stress
- Suppressed emotions
- Feeling angry for long periods
- Experiencing an intense, emotional situation for an extended period
- Being in relationships where you feel emotionally drained, unhappy, aggrieved, or resentful
- When you are unable to get over or resolve a deep emotional pain
- Low blood sugar
- Caffeine consumption
- Unhealthy diet
- Consumption of refined carbohydrates
- Lack of exercise
- Alcohol consumption
- Nutrient and vitamin deficiencies, especially B complex, calcium and magnesium
- Adrenal exhaustion
- Thyroid disorders

Unhealed emotional injuries affect us deeply, impacting every cell in our body, draining and shattering the spirit. Anger, fear, and worry can create a stress reaction that can weaken the immune system, incapacitating its ability to fight off diseases and defend the body from viruses or potentially damaging foreign substances that might enter the bloodstream. This is why emotional stresses are often the precursor to diseases. When we don't address our unresolved mental and emotional issues, we experience a variety of health problems.

The causes and impact of anxiety are as individual as

the people who suffer from it. Sometimes the symptoms will slam you like a freight train; other times, they'll develop gradually over time. Sometimes the symptoms will come and go; other times, they'll be constant. Sometimes the symptoms are mild and easy to manage; other times, they are severe and incapacitating.

How anxiety symptoms manifest often depends on the individual's coping skills. Our coping mechanism comes from the health of our adrenal glands, which regulate our stress response. When the body has experienced a stressful situation for a lengthy period, it can overwork and exhaust the adrenals, disrupting their functions and weakening them.

> *"Illnesses do not come upon us out of the blue. They are developed from small daily sins against Nature. When enough sins have accumulated, illnesses will suddenly appear."*
> *Hippocrates*

The sympathetic nervous system stimulates the adrenal glands to release stress hormones. The constant demand on these glands can lead to feelings of nervous exhaustion and being emotionally drained. We often call this feeling *burnout*.

The adrenal glands, also known as suprarenal glands, are located on top of each kidney. About the size of a walnut, these tiny glands play a crucial role in the overall health of the human body. They are composed of two sections: the adrenal cortex and the adrenal medulla. They regulate various processes and make many vital hormones. In addition to helping the body respond to stress, they regulate blood pressure, help control blood sugar, produce steroid hormones cortisol and aldosterone (aldosterone helps control blood pressure), and sex steroid hormones estrogen, progesterone, and testosterone, as well as other hormones that contribute to overall health.

Cortisol helps regulate the metabolism. High stress levels can increase cortisol production, which in turn may lower immune response, elevate blood pressure, disrupt blood serum glucose levels, and diminish serotonin levels, which can result in weight gain. Serotonin is a mood-regulating hormone that

Carolyn's Story

My earliest memories of feeling anxious go back to elementary school. I remember being very shy and going to school made me feel uneasy. I also began experiencing migraine headaches and even heart palpitations at some point. Fortunately, my heart palpitations stopped but my migraines continued from childhood into my college years.

It was in those college years that I found it extremely stressful to balance work and school at the same time, along with everything else in my life. I would say this was around the time that anxiety started to affect the quality of my sleep profoundly. I wasn't able to sleep at night. I would struggle to feel energized during the day. I was tired all the time but couldn't fall asleep. I felt restless and exhausted.

I was tired of feeling tired, so I started to research natural remedies for stress and anxiety. It was then when I decided to see a doctor of natural medicine. The doctor helped me understand my body's reaction to anxiety and stress that I was feeling for many years. The doctor recommended a variety of herbs and supplements that support the adrenal glands and reduce stress. After taking them regularly, I have finally seen a reduction of anxiety and stress. These herbal remedies have helped me cope with feelings of tiredness and anxiousness. They have helped my body attain quality sleep and feel at ease throughout the day, and I don't get migraines anymore.

Natural herbs and remedies have made a significant improvement in my quality of life. Thanks to a holistic approach, my anxiety and stress are under control. I would recommend anyone seeking help with anxiety and stress to consider natural herbs and remedies as a healthy alternative.

helps balance us emotionally; it helps us feel less nervous, more relaxed and energetic, and focused. When the adrenals are out of balance, they can disrupt the entire normal body rhythm, negatively impact the immune system, slow wound healing, cause thinning hair and weight gain, and more. The hormones I've just listed are produced by the outer part of the adrenal glands called the adrenal cortex.

Epinephrine (or adrenaline) is one of the major hormones of the sympathetic nervous system. This is the hormone released by the adrenal glands when we experience abrupt stress, fear, or shock. It increases blood sugar, heart rate, blood pressure, sweating, and shortness of breath. The adrenal glands regulate the body's stress response through the secretion of epinephrine and norepinephrine. These two hormones are produced primarily by the adrenal medulla, which is the inner part of the adrenal glands.

The special role of hormones in anxiety

Hormone imbalances can be both a cause and a result of anxiety. They affect bodily functions that are directly connected to the nervous system and the endocrine system.

Hormones are biochemical messengers that the endocrine glands, like the adrenals and the gonads, make and release into the bloodstream. For example, let's say a woman has a hormonal imbalance because her ovaries are not producing enough female hormones. At the same time, she's experiencing high stress because of life issues. This woman is going to be running on empty and is likely to experience a lot of anxiety symptoms and even panic attacks. Why? Because the adrenal glands serve as the backup for when the body needs female hormones by making small amounts of female hormones.

Stress exhausts and depletes the adrenal glands so they can't function properly.

The adrenal glands are connected to and in charge of stress management through a signal from the pituitary gland, which controls the adrenal glands. The pituitary gland, like the adrenal glands, is part of the endocrine system. The moment the brain senses stress, fear, and anger, it sends a message to the pituitary gland through the hypothalamus. This signal is a hormone called corticotropin-releasing hormone (CRH). The message activates the release of adrenocorticotropic hormone (ACTH), which will cause the adrenal glands to produce epinephrine/adrenaline and cortisol.

Epinephrine is essential for a robust cardiovascular

ENDOCRINE SYSTEM

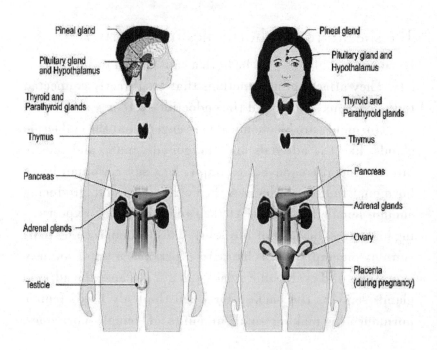

system. It helps strengthen the heart so it can beat more powerfully, diverting blood to tissues in times of stress and anxiety. That's why, when a person is experiencing intense stress or a panic attack, the heart rate, blood pressure, and even blood sugar levels are elevated. In other words, the body is getting ready for an intense action or commotion.

Cortisol, known as the stress hormone, has many functions. When it comes to anxiety, cortisol's impact includes helping the body deal with stressful situations, reducing inflammation, and increasing blood sugar, which delivers more energy and improves the brain's use of glucose.

To help explain the many processes that take place in the body when we are experiencing an anxiety attack, the

STRESS RESPONSE

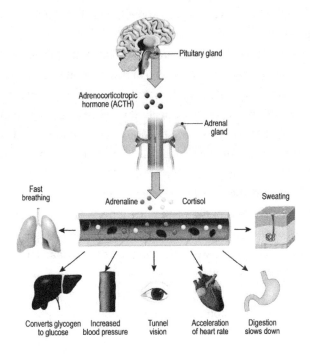

illustration on page 29 shows the steps the human body takes when it encounters stress. The illustration on page 28 shows

Jeff's Story

The first time I experienced anxiety, I was in my late teens. At the time, I had no idea what was happening to me. The roots of my anxiety went back to my childhood.

When we moved to America, my world changed dramatically. I was eight years old, didn't speak English, and felt like I didn't fit in. The pressure was tremendous, and it took a significant toll.

When I was twenty-one and getting married, I had a major breakdown. I couldn't breathe right, couldn't think straight, and was crying. I felt overwhelmed and didn't want to speak with anyone—I just wanted to sleep everything away. I didn't know I was suffering from anxiety.

Somehow I managed to survive that phase in my life, but I never understood why I was so anxious about things that should be easy for me to handle.

Years later, when I was in my forties, I started to feel some unusual sensations, including shortness of breath, tightness in my chest, heart palpitations, and confusion. I also felt claustrophobic. Even though I managed to struggle through the feelings, they were happening often enough that I became concerned that I was having heart problems. After some tests, I was told that my heart was healthy, but I was suffering from anxiety. My family doctor prescribed medication and suggested I see a counselor.

After several months of therapy for anxiety and depression, I began to understand that anxiety and panic attacks I suffered back when I was twenty-one were affecting me again. I was introduced to natural anxiety remedies that included diet, exercise, and the right kind of supplements. It took effort, but I was finally able to manage my anxiety. My symptoms disappeared, and I am enjoying life more fully.

the glands that make up the endocrine system (a group of glands that manufactures hormones) in males and females.

The adrenal glands become exhausted under a variety of circumstances, including:

- A poor diet high in refined sugars and lacking in nutrients
- A continual production of cortisol
- High consumption of caffeine
- Lack of sleep
- High or prolonged stress
- Poorly functioning pituitary gland

When the pituitary gland is not functioning well, it may not communicate effectively with the adrenals and their function may decline. The body attempts to compensate for exhausted adrenal glands, which puts pressure on all body systems because the other glands and organs must modify their normal functions to accommodate the added demand. In other words, they rescue the adrenals so body balance can be maintained. But by doing this, these systems will start to weaken over time as well, and that's how other illnesses may start someplace else in the body.

Fatigued adrenal glands create inexplicable, frustrating symptoms. For example, you may feel tired and sleepy, no matter how much sleep you get. Or you may have trouble falling asleep or waking up. You may need caffeine to get through the day but be unable to sleep at night. You may experience salt or sugar cravings, have dark circles under your eyes, feel anxious and/or depressed, have a low sex drive, poor circulation, and even low blood pressure. Some of these symptoms happened to Carolyn, whose story is on page 26.

Who gets anxiety?

Anyone can be susceptible to anxiety. It strikes males and females at any age, from child to adult to senior.

We can feel anxious as early as our time in the womb because the child feels the stress of the mother. Children and teenagers may feel anxious due to stress at home, at school,

Michele's Story

There was a time when I was unsuccessfully trying to deal with an enormous amount of stress. External factors were causing me a great deal of anxiety, but I didn't know that was what I was feeling. I was drowning in my head. I was in the process of buying my first home, planning my wedding, and managing a major job change at work. I couldn't focus on one task long enough to complete anything I needed to do. I was frustrated because the work I needed to do was piling up but I was too anxious to finish anything. I was overwhelmed and couldn't see any relief in sight. I felt ashamed and scared to tell anyone about my struggles. I thought I had to handle all of it on my own.

Finally, I opened up to a trusted coworker. I am so thankful that she told me it was okay to need help and seek that help. She did not dismiss my anxiety or tell me to get over it; she was supportive and understanding.

Thanks to my friend's encouragement, I went to my doctor. The anxiety medication she prescribed helped reduce the time I spent worrying and allowed me to focus on what I needed to do. I took the medication for a few months until I got past the situations that were so overwhelming. Then, under my doctor's supervision, I slowly weaned myself off the medication as I learned better coping techniques to manage my stress and anxiety. If you are dealing with any mental illness, let me tell you what my friend told me: It's okay to need and get help!

and elsewhere. Some anxiety symptoms youngsters exhibit include fear, nervousness, tension, quietness, isolation, nail-biting, irritability, sleep issues, sadness, and behavioral changes like anger, frustration, and guilt. Children may also develop separation anxiety, where they are nervous, sad, and fearful when they are apart from loved ones.

From my own experience with kids, I have seen that anxiety often starts at home. Monitor your stress levels because your children can sense when you are stressed, no matter how good of an act you put on, and they're affected by it. I've seen kids from high-stress homes where the parent or parents are extremely controlling and demanding. The parents' expectations and behaviors can create frustration for the child who feels unable to explain or express himself. That frustration builds and can eventually turn into anxiety and depression.

> *"Just as food causes chronic disease, it can be the most powerful cure."*
> Hippocrates

Children who consume a diet high in refined sugars and sodium with few green vegetables and fruits are also at increased risk for anxiety. When a child's or even an adult's diet consists primarily of sugary cereal or pancakes and syrup for breakfast, chicken nuggets or burgers and fries for lunch, and pizza or mac and cheese for dinner, they are an anxiety attack waiting to happen. Anyone consuming that kind of diet is going to feel fatigued, unfocused, absent-minded, and hyperactive. They're also likely to suffer from sleep disturbances like nightmares or night terrors.

Regardless of age, the body—particularly the brain and nervous systems—requires good food to function properly. Food is the body's fuel. If you feed your body low quality, cheap fuel, it runs poorly.

Seniors may develop anxiety as they age because they may find themselves alone and unable to take care of themselves. Leaving their homes to move to assisted living or nursing facilities can also trigger anxiety. On the opposite end of the age spectrum, teenagers and young adults dealing with all the pressures of growing up and coming of age may become overwhelmed, resulting in anxiety attacks.

Stress, frustration, and confusion are common emotions for people with autism, and these feelings can lead to anxiety. I could go on, but my point is: Anyone can suffer from anxiety for any reason. There is no shame in it. If you or someone you care about is feeling or exhibiting symptoms of anxiety, be proactive in dealing with it. Remember, anxiety mimics a range of physical ailments. You need to be sure, for example, that your chest pains are anxiety and not a heart attack, so see a doctor to confirm that your symptoms are anxiety and what your best course of action is.

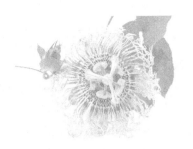

Chapter 4

How to Manage Anxiety Naturally

There is no magic pill for anxiety. Because it comes in many forms and affects people in a variety of ways, it requires a variety of treatments. Especially if you don't know the source of it, managing anxiety can be a daunting and difficult task—but don't give up, because it's doable. Because so many herbs and vitamins can provide relief from anxiety, it can be challenging and draining to find the combination that will work for you. It's also essential to discover the underlying reason for your anxiety; if you don't, any treatment is only going to be a band-aid.

In some cases, identifying and dealing with the source of your anxiety may eliminate the need for any additional treatment. Take an objective look at your life and do a thorough analysis of:

- Your stress levels in all your environments—home,

work, and elsewhere
- Your lifestyle, health, hormone levels, and current situation, including relationships
- Your diet, exercise, and sleep habits
- Recent life changes and events
- Unresolved long-term issues
- Your emotions

One way you can find relief from anxiety is by writing down everything you are feeling and everything that's bothering you. Or you can talk about it to someone you trust. This will help you release everything you are holding inside. Releasing your emotions can be very healing. Another thing to do is confront your fears. When I confronted my fears, I realized things were not really as bad as I thought. The fear was only significant in my imagination. By confronting my fears, I learned how to cope and handle those emotions.

Use the worksheet in Appendix IV as a guide. As you work through this analysis, remember that emotions are powerful. They can alter how glands and organs function. They can depress the immune system, increase blood pressure, and cause stress, so don't dismiss them. This analysis will make a huge difference in how quickly and how well you'll get relief from your anxiety.

Some processes need to take place before you can begin to restore imbalances and heal any damage to your nervous system, immune system, and adrenal glands done by these situations. Unless the adrenal glands are restored, it doesn't matter what else we do or take—anxiety will continue to affect us.

To achieve complete healing, you need a body/mind/spirit connection. When you have that, the healing pathways will open, and the body can synchronize with what's going on internally and externally. Negative emotions can interfere and block these healing pathways, disconnecting the body from the soul and the mind. Some negative emotions are:

- Anger
- Anxiousness
- Blame
- Depression
- Envy
- Fear
- Frustration
- Grief
- Guilt
- Hate
- Helplessness
- Hopelessness
- Impatience
- Jealousy
- Loneliness
- Mistrust
- Nervousness
- Resentment
- Sadness
- Shame
- Worry

Our bodies need to be in harmony so our systems and organs can communicate and conduct their normal and constant functions. I believe that happiness and positive mental thinking are the best ways to commence healing and maintain steady health. When we are happy and when we laugh, it brings joy, contentment, and gratification to our soul. Happiness and joyful feelings can heal us from within. They mend us inside; they remove sadness and restore unsettled inner emotions. In turn, this allows our bodies to reconnect and our systems and organs to synchronize so health can return. The old saying that laughter is the best medicine is true.

Happiness and positive mental thinking are of supreme importance when trying to heal from any illness, especially anxiety, because the mind is a powerful instrument that either supports or destroys. We must choose to be positive and keep going, to not allow negative thinking and emotions to take hold, because once they do, it will be very hard to recover. If we tell ourselves consciously or subconsciously that we can't heal, we can't cope, we're not going to get better, we can't do it, or there's no way out, that's the message the body will receive and it will respond accordingly. Also, what we reflect is what we are going to attract. What you are constantly imagining is what the universe will give you.

> *"The secret of health for both mind and body is not to mourn for the past, nor to worry about the future, but to live the present moment wisely and earnestly."*
> *Siddhartha Gautama*

Instead, surround yourself with friends and family, with people who support you and make you happy. Do activities you enjoy. Consistently put yourself in positive situations so the grief and anxiety can disappear and your body and mind can heal. I understand this may be easier said than done, but you must make the effort. We don't get well—or accomplish anything!—by sitting down and waiting for something to happen to us; we have to get up and *make* it happen, no matter how easy or difficult it might be. Determination and belief are powerful. Once you have resolved that you *can* help yourself, that you *are* going to find answers, and that you *will* get better, you will find the strength and resources to make it happen.

This is where the connection between the body and the mind needs to happen. You must retrain your brain to turn negative thoughts into positive ones. When you have a negative thought, immediately reject it. Say to yourself, "I don't believe this thought is real. It will not happen. I'm going to be okay no matter how I'm feeling right now. This thought is only because of anxiety, and I don't accept it." If you believe it, your inner sense of awareness will believe it, too, and then your body will accept it and respond to it.

One thing I learned from my struggle with anxiety is that worry never resolved any of my concerns and fears, worry never changed the situation, and whether I worried or not, the problem was still there. So why worry?

For example, if I'm running late for something, can I change being late by worrying and fretting? No. I'm late, and I'm going to be late no matter what I do, so why worry? Instead, I find a positive way to deal with the situation.

When you're worried about something, take a step back and ask yourself what you can accomplish by worrying. The answer will always be nothing. Chase the worrisome emotions away by reminding yourself of this each time those thoughts creep into your mind.

The power of negative thinking

Constant negative thoughts, negative feelings, negative behaviors, and a negative environment produce a vibration that upset the body's chemistry, including hormonal function. This can affect every cell of the human body. With a negative mental attitude, we are harming ourselves, exhausting our glands and organs, and creating health issues.

Too many people are walking around empty, unfulfilled, seeking material things they think will make them happy, then looking for even more when what they have isn't enough. They neglect their souls for material things. Their minds are so cluttered with negative thoughts and burdened with stress and fatigue that they don't have room for good thoughts and positive feelings. This attachment to negative emotions, habits, ideas, and attitudes harms them physically and mentally.

Like hormone imbalances, negative thinking can be both the cause and the result of an anxiety attack, which is why it's so critical to understand and address how our thought processes impact our emotional and physical health. When someone suffers an anxiety attack, they usually feel unraveled, derailed, and out of control. Their body is doing things on its own, and they can't do things they want to do. They feel insecure, which opens the door to negative thoughts and more anxiety.

By being positive in every situation, no matter how difficult it is for us at the moment, we allow our body to be infused with the right kind of natural chemicals, and that gives us the chance to heal properly. Anxiety disconnects body, mind, and spirit. Unless we ground ourselves, we are not going to feel whole and complete again.

Healing the mind and body

We need to take control of our thoughts and emotions because only then can we experience a real sense of well-being, and when we do, we will be able to combat anxiety. Healing comes from within by nurturing your spirit. God made our bodies to be self-healing. It is the connection that exists in our inner conscience, the innate ability that we were born with, that allows our body to mend. To restore itself, the body must harmonize with good feelings, thoughts, and actions—all elements of a healthy mind. And a healthy mind does well to the body just as a healthy body does well to the mind.

So how do you do it? Through personal experience and research, I've found a customized combination of healing therapies, vitamins, herbs, and flower essences work together to help us heal from anxiety. These therapies and supplements can produce a profound inner restoration, producing changes so that the body can balance itself, just the way nature intended to be.

Some of the ways the body may start to reconnect and restore itself are by deep breathing, visualization, exercising, massage, meditation, yoga, music, and prayer. When the body can start regrouping and rearranging itself internally, the mind, body, and spirit can bond and keep us in balance. There are groups of flower essences and herbs that play an important part in supporting the body's inborn natural healing process; they're explained in Appendix I and II.

Here are some natural ways through which we may find relief and support:

Sleep. The most important part of healing is sleep. Sleep restores the body. It's essential for a healthy immune system and nervous system. Getting a good night's rest allows your mind to regroup and rid itself of anxious thoughts and or accumulated stress. While we sleep, the body is at work to keep us healthy by repairing cells, restoring energy, and maintaining healthful brain function. During sleep, the brain detoxifies and rearranges and stores information so we are fresh when we wake up. This is why when we don't sleep well or an adequate amount, we often don't feel like talking or listening the next day because our brains and bodies are overloaded with unwanted information and toxins from the day before.

Reduce caffeine and alcohol consumption. Caffeine is a stimulant that will energize your body for a short time. While alcohol sometimes feels like a stimulant, it's actually a depressant. Excessive caffeine consumption can make us edgy and nervous. Excessive alcohol consumption leads to intoxication. Caffeine and alcohol are both addictive, and the more we consume, the more we need. When we reduce or eliminate caffeine and alcohol, our body adjusts, and we can feel energized without these substances.

Support and heal the adrenal glands. One of the functions of the adrenal glands is to regulate stress. When the adrenal glands are out of balance or depleted, they can't do their job. If you're exhausted and experiencing stress and anxiety, some of the symptoms that your adrenal glands need help include: fatigue no matter how much you sleep; restless sleep; dark circles under the eyes; quivering tongue; shakiness; emotional sensitivity; disturbing dreams that wake you up at all hours of the night; nightmares; night sweats; hot palms of the hands and soles of feet. You can restore your adrenal glands by getting the right amount of sleep; taking B vitamins, vitamin C, and minerals; drinking quality water; taking a good adrenal support compound that can deliver nutrients specifically formulated to nourish and energize the adrenals; and with adaptogenic herbs like ashwagandha, Korean ginseng, eleuthero roots, Schisandra, skullcap or wood betony.

Flower remedy for emotional healing. This is one of the best ways to calm and restore a restless mind and body because these liquid extracts address deep issues of emotional well-being. An English doctor named Dr. Eduard Bach discovered flower remedies in the 1930s. Dr. Bach said, "Seek the outstanding mental conflict in the person, give him the remedy that will overcome that conflict and all the hope and encouragement you can, then the virtue within him will itself do all the rest." He also said, "True healing involves the very base of the cause of suffering. Therefore, no effort directed to the body alone could do more than superficially repair damage. Heal people of their emotional unhappiness, allow them to be happy, and they will become well." If mental and emotional conflicts and unhappiness are not resolved, we will be unable to heal, no matter how many things we take for it. Dr. Bach's flower remedies are so effective because they harmonize us internally, reconnecting and mending our inner being, and creating equilibrium from within.

"Every human being is the author of his own health or disease."
Sivananda

Minerals. Minerals—especially magnesium, known as "the relaxer"—calm the nerves, relax the mind, and soothe the nervous system, all of which helps us get more restful sleep. A magnesium deficiency can agitate the nervous system, making a person anxious, fidgety, edgy, nervous, restless, afraid, and worried. Women may experience different symptoms, such as changes in appetite and moods. Eating organic food high in magnesium may help balance the deficiency, or you may need magnesium in tablet form. A combination of minerals that includes calcium and magnesium may be a better choice than magnesium alone because minerals work better together. Some magnesium-rich foods are nuts, whole grains, fruits and vegetables, yellow cornmeal, and wheat germ.

Vitamin B complex. B vitamins support the nervous

system and brain activities.

Omega-3 fatty acids. Omega-3 and 6 deficiencies are somehow connected with anxiety, perhaps because essential fatty acids provide nutrition to the nervous system and the brain. The body needs good fats. If we consume mostly saturated and unhealthy fats, we disrupt the proper ratio of omega-3, 6, and 9, which can contribute to unfavorable health conditions.

Nutrition. What we eat is of utmost importance to the overall well-being of our body. We often find ourselves eating too much of the wrong things and not enough of the right things. This creates nutrient deficiencies that not only deplete and disrupt brain function but also alter gland and organ functions, resulting in unwanted ailments and conditions and hormone imbalances.

Herbs. Herbs play an important role in our overall health and healing. When it comes to anxiety, there are a few that can be of tremendous assistance because they help promote calmness, decrease nervousness, and help with sleep. Some of these herbs are passionflower, valerian root, and hops, which are botanical herbs known historically for their ability to bring relaxation and calmness into some one's life as well as aiding sleep. For better results, find a combination of them. A list of herbal combinations and other herbs beneficial for stress and anxiety is in Appendix II.

Address your hormones. When someone is suffering from anxiety, one of the first things to do is to check their hormone levels. Hormones can completely change how we feel from one moment to another. We might have a hormone imbalance and not know it. For example, low estrogen can cause anxiety, hot flashes, fast heart rate, heart palpitations, dizziness, depression, headaches, insomnia, and more. I have seen people suffering from anxiety for a long time only to find that their hormones were out of balance. Chronic stress and any of the other causes of anxiety we discussed in Chapter Three can create hormone imbalances. While women are more prone to hormone imbalances, especially when they are going through perimenopause or menopause, the need to check hormones is not exclusive to females; men should have their hormones checked, as well.

Stress management. Managing stress is important even when you're not dealing with anxiety, and it's critical when you are. Chronic stress is like a bucket that's filling up with water; when it gets full to the brim, just a drop can make it overflow. That's when the body becomes overwhelmed, and even everyday noises can be startling or cause anxiousness—and pretty soon, you're in a full-blown anxiety episode because the body can't cope. Of course, most of the things we do daily have a degree of stress associated with them. One solution is to take more time

> *"And may we ever have gratitude in our hearts that the great Creator in all His glory has placed the herbs in the field for our healing."*
> Dr. Edward Bach

to enjoy what really matters in our lives and stop trying to multi-task. By doing that, we will have a deeper sense of satisfaction and appreciation for everything we do and every moment we experience, which will ease our stress. When we focus on one thing at a time, we're able to grasp more, we're more productive, and we're more satisfied. When we try to multi-task, all we're doing is dedicating less time to each task or conversation. Part of our brain is distracted, so we often don't end up doing our best and things don't get completed as they should, which creates more stress.

Music. Because gentle music can calm, soothe, and relax

our minds, it can bring a sense of happiness, therefore helping in calming down anxiety.

Aromatherapy. In ancient times, some essential oils were known for their soothing and relaxing effects. The fragrance of these oils may help reduce stress, alleviate insomnia, and improve concentration. Some of these essential oils are lavender, bergamot, Roman chamomile, frankincense, orange, and ylang ylang.

> *"Those who do not find time every day for health must sacrifice a lot of time one day for illness."*
> *Father Sebastian Kneipp*

Forgiveness. When you forgive, you heal yourself. You gain an inner sense of freedom and peace. Forgiving allows us to move on with life. It untangles us from anything holding us back emotionally, purifying our hearts and spirits as it frees the path to renewal and a fresh life. When we're filled with anger and resentment at someone else, we don't harm the target of our emotions; we harm ourselves. Forgiving cleanses and refreshes the heart and mind, it restores, it makes us whole, and it mends relationships. Forgiving brings good energy; let it circulate through your whole being, healing and liberating you.

Yoga. Yoga is calming to the mind, restorative to the muscles, relaxing, and helps bring balance and peace.

Massage. Massages can be very soothing, relaxing, and invigorating. They help destress tensed muscles, calm the mind, and ease related issues that can accompany anxiety.

Exercise. Physical exercise can help release unwanted stress. Even a brisk walk will help you breathe cleansing fresh air as it refreshes your mind. While you're walking or doing any other form of exercise, focus on positive thoughts and affirmations. Of course, check with your doctor before beginning a new exercise program.

Deep breathing. One of the fastest ways to calm an anxious heart is deep breathing. Focusing on your breathing distracts your brain from whatever is causing stress and gives you a chance to let go of your anxiety.

Visualization. We all go through times we wish we could avoid, but we can't—that's life. When you find yourself in those moments, pause and see yourself after it has passed. Visualize what your life will look like when the difficult time is over, and you'll find it easier to deal with the present. But visualization is more than a stress-management tool. Take the time to clearly and vividly visualize what you want in life, where you want to be, who you want to be with, and what you want to change in your current situation. Let your visualizations keep you on track to achieving your dreams.

Meditation. Meditation helps reconnect our body with our mind and soul. It brings peace, order, and serenity into a restless and disturbed mind. Meditation is calming to the mind; it helps calm the mental chatter and the neurotic thoughts that we can experience when suffering from anxiety. Meditation can also be done by meditating on God's Word.

Pray. Praying and grounding ourselves by trusting that the Lord has everything under His control is a big part of healing. Turning our anxiety, worries, and burdens over to the Lord and believing He can help us heal gives us rest.

The Choice is Yours

We are in charge of our health. We are responsible for what we put into our bodies—not just supplements, but food. The choices we make will have a direct impact on our health, so we must not depend on anyone else to make decisions for us.

A common nutritional mistake is either consuming too little protein or too much protein and fats. Insufficient protein will create hormonal and thyroid imbalances. The body needs protein to make hormones and enzymes and for building and repairing tissue. Protein is a vital component of bones, blood, cartilage, hair, muscles, nails, and skin. The body also needs carbohydrates and fats.

The body breaks protein down into amino acids, which are necessary for many body functions and processes. There are twenty amino acids our bodies need. They function together in an exclusive balance and any disruption will affect organs, glands, and the brain. We produce eleven of them, which are called nonessential amino acids. The other nine are the essential amino acids the body can't produce, which must be supplied by the protein we consume daily. Because our body doesn't store amino acids, they need to be part of our daily diet. The brain requires certain amino acids like arginine, histidine, tyrosine and tryptophan to properly syn-thesize neurotransmitters and neuromodulators.

Too much animal protein can put pressure on the kidneys, increasing uric acid levels and lowering the body's capacity to absorb calcium. This can cause kidney stones. New research also suggests that too much animal protein may increase the risk of fatty liver disease.

Our bodies also need phosphorous. There are two types: One for the brain and the other for bones. The phosphorous needed by the brain comes from animal products (meat, milk, egg yolk, fish, and fish roe) and the phosphorous needed for bones comes from plants, nuts, and seeds (almonds, rice bran, wheat bran, wheat germ, pumpkin, sunflower and squash seeds).

It is vital to understand how our bodies function and the

nutrition necessary to properly fuel them if we are to maintain optimum health.

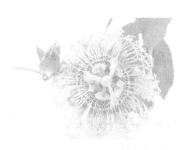

Chapter 5

How Faith Helps Heal Anxiety

When you suffer from anxiety, it's normal to feel alone, to feel like you're the only one going through this. You look around and it seems like everyone else is doing well, living happy lives, and you are the only one struggling with all-consuming turmoil. It's a burden that won't release you. You might feel that God has abandoned you, that He is not listening to you, and that you are all alone in your suffering.

In Joshua 1:9, God says, "Have I not commanded you? Be strong and courageous. Do not be afraid; do not be discouraged, for the Lord your God will be with you wherever you go." Deuteronomy 31:6 says, "Be strong and courageous, do not be afraid or terrified because of them, for the Lord your God goes with you; He will never leave you nor forsake you."

I know it's easy for me to say this, to give you Bible verses, and to tell you what to do when I'm not the one currently going through anxious moments or a full-blown anxiety attack. I also know it's hard to believe and have faith when you're suffering. It's hard to know that God is next to you, listening and helping you even when you don't feel Him. I also understand that even though anxiety is different for everyone, it's still so powerful that there may be no room for other feelings or for anything to enter and help us. I know this because that's how I felt. And even though I knew how to help someone else, I was too frightened, too full of fear, too shattered to help myself.

"Faith is not belief without proof, but trust without reservation."

Elton Trueblood

If that's where you are now, know this: You are not crazy, you are not losing your mind.

You have a problem—a problem that can be managed using the techniques we discussed in Chapter Four. Let's talk about combining those practical techniques with faith.

Believing that the Lord is near us but not getting help from Him as fast as we need it can make us ask questions like: Why isn't He helping me and answering my pleas? Did I do something to upset God? Did I sin without knowing? Why is He allowing me to suffer this way? Where is His compassion for me right now? Doesn't He know that I'm suffering?

I've asked all those questions and more. I've discovered that the answer is that we must be patient, have faith, keep believing in Him, and don't get discouraged. There is always a reason why our suffering is taking time to get resolved. I believe that He is preparing us for something greater, there is a lesson for whatever experience we're going through, and our struggles can make us stronger and better.

The Bible discusses many people who suffered. Two are Joseph and David. Joseph was mistreated and left for dead by his brothers, then was sold as a slave. He never imagined that God had a plan for him, that the reason he was going through this painful experience was because he was to save his family from a devastating famine.

David struggled with anxiety and depression as he was hunted by King Saul. But those struggles led him to write the majority of the Book of Psalms and eventually become the King of Israel. We are blessed even today by his life experiences because we can read his encouraging Psalms and poems that relate to our own difficulties.

The Apostle Paul wrote: "We were under great pressure, far beyond our ability to endure, so that we despaired of life itself. Indeed, we felt we had received the sentence of death." (2 Corinthians 1:8-9) Even though he was at such a low point in his ministry, he was still able to conquer with God's help and write most of the New Testament that we so enjoy today. Some of the greatest accomplishments have been achieved because of great pain or struggle in our lives.

How I was finally able to heal wasn't just by praying and waiting for something to happen. Yes, I prayed a lot, but it wasn't working for me. I wondered and asked God why some people were healed instantly just by asking—why not me? Why would I hear people sharing their stories of miraculous healing and I wasn't healed? I was a good person, I hadn't done anything wrong. Why was I going through this?

I spent hours asking God those questions but didn't get any answers. I was desperate. I thought I was going to be sick for the rest of my life. I felt alone because no one understood what I was going through. I felt empty, my heart was hollow, and I was afraid God wasn't there, He wasn't listening to my pleas. But I kept praying because if I didn't, I had no hope.

One night while I was praying and feeling like I was just talking to no one, I decided not to worry. It was a decision borne of desperation. I prayed: "Lord, I give up. I have tried everything that I know and can. I surrender to You. You decide if you want to heal me or take me tonight. I'm not going to fight all this anymore. I'm tired of it. Whatever you do, I will accept."

The next day was the first day I felt something was different in me, but I didn't quite know what yet. But that day, I found an answer that was the beginning of my healing with natural remedies.

I admit that when I was experiencing anxiety and the related panic attacks, I didn't think something good was going to come out of it. In fact, I didn't believe I was going to get out of it at all. I didn't believe I would get better. I didn't see the light; it was all darkness for me. I couldn't find the way out; I couldn't break the cycle I was in.

"My job is to take care of the possible and trust God with the impossible."
Ruth Bell Graham

It took a long time for me to understand it all. I felt foreign, like I was living in a bad dream. But I kept believing. Even though I didn't feel God with me, I convinced myself that He was there. I couldn't imagine otherwise.

Situations like I was in, situations full of pain and suffering, can make us ask the right questions—questions that get profound results and an understanding of what needs changing in our lives at that time. We all go through unwanted experiences in life, but it is these experiences that polish us, teach us, and train us. In my case, my experience with anxiety was preparing me to help others going through the same desperation and confusion, to help them heal physically and grow spiritually.

As you pray, be patient and trusting. Help will come, even though it might seem that it's taking a long time, and it isn't going to happen for you. Don't give up. Hang in there and wait because the answer always comes.

I mistrusted Him in my darkest moment, I questioned and disbelieved His compassion, kindness, and love for me, but in the end, I realized that God was always there for me, He has never failed me. He knows what we need and what is good for us. So, my friends, be patient and wait. Don't give up even if it has been a long time for you. You can do it. You will conquer your situation. Don't lose hope because there is always a solution.

When you're feeling anxious, remind yourself that God's help will find its way to you, in one way or another. His help may not be direct, and it may not happen immediately. He knows you're suffering and waiting for His help, but it's important to trust His timing. In my case, God's help came through relatives who helped me deal with my situation. They strengthened my beliefs, they didn't let me doubt, and they kept reminding me of His promises, and that gave me the will-power to continue trying. Be open to God working through people. Someone may give you an idea for something you can do or take to help your condition or situation, or just simply offer comforting words from the Bible or a sermon. Believing and trusting will bring you hope, peace, and calmness.

I know this because I was there. I was lost and confused about my situation. I didn't understand what was happening to me. I felt alone. At night, I worried that I was going to die because even when I finally fell asleep, the anxiety episodes would wake me up. It felt like someone was torturing and tormenting me with so many symptoms all day and all night. Most nights, I would wake up drenched in sweat and trembling from nightmares that haunted me. In those moments, I would search for God in the dark. Was He there? Did He hear me? The more I pleaded, the more distant from Him I felt. It was like someone else was controlling me. All I heard was silence, with no reassurance that everything was going to be okay. It seemed like God had abandoned me.

If you've felt this way, believe me: Help will arrive in time. Keep praying and asking. Be patient in your suffering. Don't frustrate yourself with fear and impatience. Let Him show you the way in His own time. He will.

The Apostle Peter wrote, "Cast all your anxiety on Him because He cares for you." (1 Peter 5:7) And He does! It's our own thoughts and imaginations that make us feel like He doesn't, especially when we need Him the most.

To come out of feeling abandoned by God and start feeling that you matter and that you are as special to Him as if you were the only person in the whole universe, begin by studying His Word. When we read the Bible, we feel reassured of his promises to us; we learn more about Him and how He will catch us before we collapse entirely. The reason there are so many verses in the Bible that talk about sadness, anxiety, and fear is to help us become whole again. Reading His Word will cleanse our minds from negative thoughts, fear, and worry; it will heal and calm your spirit.

When you don't feel God's presence, when you don't see any sign that your prayers are being heard, know this: You are wrong. Anxiety has a way of bringing thoughts and fears to our minds that are not true. These negative ideas exist in our imaginations, and if you were free from anxiety, you wouldn't be thinking them.

Healing Anxiety • 57

When you are thinking negative, depressing things, question your thoughts. Don't allow them to control you. Ask yourself: *Is this true? I didn't think like this before, why am I thinking this now?* The more you do this, the easier it will be to disbelieve the negative thoughts that are not real because they are coming from your anxiety.

Learn to live in the present. Don't worry about tomorrow; tomorrow will take care of itself. Focus on what is happening now, manage your feelings as they come, and soon you will be able to control your thoughts and eliminate the false fears.

I am entirely sympathetic to anyone going through a tough time. I understand how difficult it is to believe when things seem to be all wrong. I've been there—afraid, hopeless, disconnected, sure that God didn't care, feeling like I was going to die. I didn't recognize myself.

> *"Faith is taking the first step even when you don't see the whole staircase."*
> *Martin Luther King, Jr.*

When I decided to dedicate time for Him, to build a relationship with Him—not just ask for Him to do things for me, but to talk with Him and listen to Him, I began to feel different. Something majestic was returned to me. A sense of peace, of relief, even of liberation swept through my whole body. I felt protected.

It was the first step on my healing journey. I was finally free from the oppression of anxiety. Yes, I still had work to do. I still had to get my body healthy and back in balance. But it was my faith and my relationship with the Lord that made me able to do that. That's why I'm telling you to trust in Him and leave everything with Him, liberate yourself from the oppression of anxiety, open your heart to Him, get close to Him, rejoice in Him, and you, too, will experience healing.

Psalm 91

Whoever dwells in the shelter of the Most High
　will rest in the shadow of the Almighty.
I will say of the Lord, "He is my refuge and my fortress,
　my God, in whom I trust."
Surely he will save you
　from the fowler's snare
　and from the deadly pestilence.
He will cover you with his feathers,
　and under his wings you will find refuge;
　his faithfulness will be your shield and rampart.
You will not fear the terror of night,
　nor the arrow that flies by day,
nor the pestilence that stalks in the darkness,
　nor the plague that destroys at midday.
A thousand may fall at your side,
　ten thousand at your right hand,
　but it will not come near you.
You will only observe with your eyes
　and see the punishment of the wicked.
If you say, "The Lord is my refuge,"
　and you make the Most High your dwelling,
no harm will overtake you,
　no disaster will come near your tent.
For he will command his angels concerning you
　to guard you in all your ways;
they will lift you up in their hands,
　so that you will not strike your foot against a stone.
You will tread on the lion and the cobra;
　you will trample the great lion and the serpent.
"Because he loves me," says the Lord, "I will rescue him;
　I will protect him, for he acknowledges my name.
He will call on me, and I will answer him;
　I will be with him in trouble,
　I will deliver him and honor him.
With long life I will satisfy him
　and show him my salvation."

Jesus said, "Come to me, all you who are weary and burdened, and I will give you rest. Take my yoke upon you and learn from me, for I am gentle and humble in heart, and you will find rest for your souls." (Matthew 11:28-29). When God is in our lives, everything runs as it should. When we follow His will, everything is perfect, and everything falls into place. When He is in us, everything synchronizes within us.

One Psalm that always gave me strength and still does today no matter the circumstances is Psalm 91. This Psalm brought peace to my heart when I had doubts and was worried. It kept me grounded.

The Word of God is true and God does what He promises. Allow Him and His power to fill your life and control your actions and every situation you go through. Read the Bible and trust the verses that tell you how we can find help and rescue in times of oppression and desperation. Even if you don't feel it right away, don't give up. Anxiety is strong, but God is stronger.

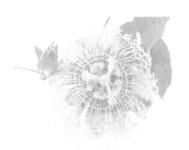

Chapter 6

Living as a Survivor

As you consider a natural approach to managing anxiety or any other ailment, begin by seeking the advice of your doctor or licensed professional healthcare provider or practitioner. This is important for several reasons: First, it will allow you to find the actual cause of your condition. Second, the treatment will be specific to your issues. Third, the recommendations will be tailored to your needs after your provider has considered all your symptoms, your overall health, various test results, the medications and supplements you are already taking, and any other relevant factors.

It's important to recognize the healing power of organic compounds. Herbs contain medicinal properties that may not be known without research, which is why it's important to consult with a professional before using natural remedies of any sort. Trained providers know the properties and contrain-dications of the herbs and supplements they recommend. For example, some herbs should only be taken for a limited time; some may not work correctly if not taken in combination with others; some may even irritate body systems and organs. Other factors a provider will consider are your body's ability to absorb supplements as well as your general state of health because sometimes the body needs to be prepared before beginning a natural remedy program. Your body's systems may need to be detoxified, rebuilt, and strengthened so that when you start, your body is ready to absorb, balance, and heal. This approach is safer for you and prevents you from wasting your money or harming yourself.

> *"A careful physician, before he attempts to administer a remedy to his patients, must investigate not only the malady of the man he wishes to cure, but also his habits when in health, and his physical constitution."*
>
> Cicero

Herbs, flower essences, and essential oils are beneficial for an array of conditions and are safe if used appropriately. Do your research and obtain the guidance of a trained healthcare professional so you can enjoy the full benefits of a natural approach without harm.

Looking back, moving forward

Though my experience with anxiety was the most diffi-cult challenge I have ever faced, I don't regret it for a moment. Anxiety struck me like lightning with an enormous force, it disabled me, it unraveled me, it shook me to my core, it took me to a dark place I had never known, full of fear and anguish.

Seemingly coming from out of nowhere, anxiety crippled me, took away my independence, and controlled me completely.

At the same time, it was an enormous gift and blessing. It brought me closer to God, strengthen my faith and trust in the Lord, and taught me how to have a relationship with Jesus. It made me a stronger, better person.

When I first started writing about anxiety, I thought my faith was strong, that I was a good person, and that was all I needed. The difference between then and now is that then I would pray and say, "Lord, you are in control. Please help me [with whatever situation I had going on]." I kept asking and asking, but I didn't feel content or reassured that my prayer would be answered. I was ruled by uncertainty.

And once the storm is over, you won't remember how you made it through, how you managed to survive. You won't even be sure whether the storm is really over. But one thing is certain. When you come out of the storm, you won't be the same person who walked in. That's what this storm's all about."

Haruki Murakami

But by studying more about trusting Him, my trust was fortified. I learned how to completely and truly rely on Him. I feel His strength from within.

I now pray and relax, knowing that everything is in His control. No matter the outcome, I don't worry. I thank Him for everything—the good and the bad.

Anxiety has also made me realize what's important in my life, to appreciate the many blessings I have, to not take anyone or anything for granted, and to treasure every minute, especially time with my family. I don't let a day go by without letting my husband and my sons know how much they mean to me and how much I love them. I don't waste time when I'm with them. We have meaningful conversations; I share with them, and I listen to what they have to say. I genuinely want to know how they are feeling and doing. And I want them to learn from my experience, to know how to be content with the present even as they are working toward their goals for the future.

Surviving anxiety has made me more patient. It's taught me to take time to listen to others sincerely. It showed me that I am vulnerable. Before my first anxiety attack, I'd never been sick. I didn't know what it was like to be sick, it never occurred to me that I would get sick, so I was shocked when it happened to me. But since then, I've learned how extraordinarily precious life is. I don't procrastinate; I won't worry. I live every day to its fullest and leave tomorrow to take care of itself. I give as much as I can, I help as many people as I can.

Anxiety has a way of changing how we think and behave. Sufferers worry more, and obsessive-compulsive behavior can manifest. I understand because I've been there.

Researching the herbs, flower essences, essential oils, and other natural ways to manage anxiety has given me a deeper understanding of how all these elements work alone and together so I can share that knowledge with those who need it.

Of course, had I not had the experience of debilitating anxiety, I would not have had the motivation to write about it so I could help others. It is my hope and prayer that you find something helpful in this book, something that will bring you relief from whatever you are going through, and that you come to understand this phase in your life and let it make you stronger and better.

I know I can't change the world, but if sharing my story and what I have learned helps someone who is navigating the difficult path of anxiety find relief, or if it helps a sufferer's loved ones help them, then the effort I put into writing this book is more than worth it.

Liberate yourself from the oppression of anxiety, allow your heart and mind to be free, allow your body to repair the damage and restore balance, and focus on knowing that life is good and the future is bright.

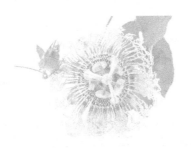

Appendix I

Flower Essences

Flower Remedies were developed by Edward Bach, an English medical doctor, homeopath, bacteriologist, and pathologist. He observed that unresolved and repressed emotions and struggles created disharmony between the mind and soul, and that these conflicts would one day lead to physical ailments. Bach believed that a person's ability to heal physically was connected to the soundness of their emotional state.

As part of his research into vaccines, he began studying plants and flowers, concluding that various flowers have a vibrational design that matches the soul frequency of the human energy field and can help restore our inner emotions and imbalances by harmonizing our spirit and soul. Bach discovered a method of extracting the healing properties of flowers through a distillation process. This creates a vibrational infusion that contributes to emotional healing.

In explaining his principles for using plants, Dr. Bach wrote: "Plants are of three types. The first group is relatively below that of a man in their evolution; of such are the primitive varieties, the seaweeds, the cactus, the dodder, etc. A second class is on the same relative scale as man, which are harmless and may be used as food. But there is a third group relatively high or higher than average mankind. Of these we must choose our remedies, for they have been given the power to heal and to bless. These plants are there to extend a helping hand to man in those dark hours of forgetfulness, when he loses sight of his divinity, and allow the clouds of fear or pain to obscure his vision."

The thirty-eight flower essence remedies he formulated are still available today. You may be familiar with Rescue Remedy, one of his most famous blends. This is a combination of five individual flowers designed to help reactivate the body's self-healing ability, providing immediate effects by restoring and calming in stressful and traumatic situations.

This section includes the flower essences known to support healing for anxiety, fear, stress, and grief. It lists the flower, the emotional/psychological characteristics and physical/general indicators of someone who may benefit from the essence, and the outcome that may result.

Using flower essence remedies is simple. You can add them to water or another beverage, or put drops under your tongue. You can take them individually or in combination with other flower essences. To determine which essence or combination of essences you need, review the information below or take the self-help assessment at the end of this appendix. A natural health practitioner can also help determine which flower is best for you.

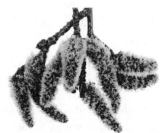

Aspen *(Popucus tremula)*

For the feeling of anxiety, worry, and inexplicable fears.

Emotional/Psychological Characteristics: Fear of the dark; fear that something terrible is going to happen; afraid of the unknown or for no reason; frequent panic attacks; nightmares and afraid to go back to sleep; imagining frightening things; can't tell the difference between reality and fantasy. In children, being afraid of the dark and having to have a light on, or fear of a monster in the closet or under the bed.

Physical/General Indicators: Fearful, tremors, exhaustion, feebleness, talking while asleep, sleepwalking.

Positive Outcome: Able to detect reality from illusion; feeling safe and self-confident; less fearful and strong sense of security; more at ease and peaceful.

~~~

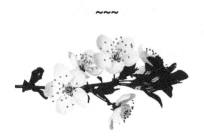

Cherry Plum *(Prunus cerasifera)*

For people who are afraid that they might do something they can't control, who fear losing control over themselves and their thoughts.

Emotional/Psychological Characteristics: Worry about losing self-control and giving into urges; fear of doing something terrible; fear of breaking down; fear of uncontrollable thoughts; confused and unable to explain feelings; suicidal.

Physical/General Indicators: Lost in thoughts; nervous; distressed; dejected; explosive in rage; tantrums in children.

Positive Outcome: Rational thoughts; relaxed and in more harmony with oneself; able to deal with emotions calmly.

~~~

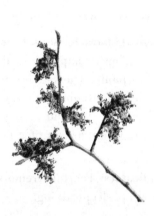

Elm (Ulmus procera)

For those who feel inundated and overtaken by their everyday tasks; find it too difficult to cope with tasks, which leaves them dis-illusioned and unhappy.

Emotional/Psychological Characteristics: Feeling that responsi-bilities are becoming too much to handle; feeling tired and being burdened by responsibilities; feeling overwhelmed and drained; has moments of insecurity; lacks strength to continue with tasks.

Physical/General Indicators: Doubtful; depressed; fatigued; hopeless.

Positive Outcome: Positive and confident with the ability to achieve tasks; reassured of the ability to handle responsibilities; more able and receptive to asking for and receiving help.

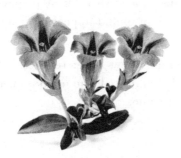

Gentian (Gentiana amarella)

For negative people, pessimists, for those who always see the negative in everything.

Emotional/Psychological Characteristics: Lack of trust in everything they do and in others, negative thoughts, often feeling discouraged.

Physical/General Indicators: Gloomy, depressed, unmotivated, unhappy.

Positive Outcome: Energized, eager and self-assured, more trusting and able to cope with obstacles and pessimism in a positive way.

~~~

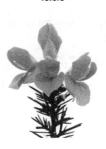

Gorse (Ulex europaeus)

For those who feel defeated and hopeless; who have given up.

Emotional/Psychological Characteristics: Exhausted, drained with no energy to keep going; insecure; no strength to try again; no hope for change; deep sorrow and discontent; heartbroken..

Physical/General Indicators: No interest in new ideas and would rather stay in that state; pallid appearance; no motivation; complete gloom.

Positive Outcome: Finds new hope; realizes that there might be other possibilities; feels uplifted; the mind is energized; more confident in a positive outcome.

~~~

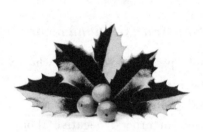

Holly (Ilex aquifolium)

For people who are jealous, envious, insecure, suspicious, hateful, and vengeful; who lack love.

Emotional/Psychological Characteristics: Suspicious, filled with jealousy, animosity, envy, and resentment.

Physical/General Indicators: Vengeful, bad temperament, intolerant, and confrontational.

Positive Outcome: Unselfish, feels calmer and thinking is positive, feels more open to love and kind toward others, expresses gratefulness.

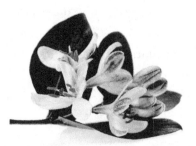

Honeysuckle (Lonicera caprifolium)

For people who live in the past; for the nostalgic; for those who live yearning for previous life experiences.

Emotional/Psychological Characteristics: Dwells in the past; doesn't see the good in the present; feels like nothing is as good as it used to be; negative about present life circumstances; discontent; negative future outlook; unable to accept changes.

Physical/General Indicators: Conversations most often are about the past, not interested in the present, stuck in the memories of the past.

Positive Outcome: More able to accept changes, capable of seeing the positive about present life, accepting of present circumstances, willing to move on from past memories and live in the present.

~~~

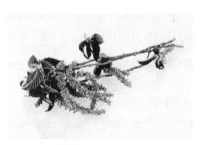

Hornbeam (Carpinus betulus)

For people who are exhausted, weary, and need strengthening.

Emotional/Psychological Characteristics: Indecisive, doubtful, unfulfilled with job routine, unhappy, and overburdened; feels mentally exhausted.

Physical/General Indicators: Drained, low energy, overweight, doesn't feel like doing any activities or anything taxing.

Positive Outcome: Energetic, keen to do activities, happier, revitalized.

~~~

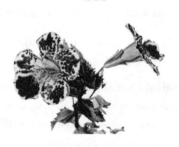

Mimulus (*Mimulus guttatus*)

For people who have a fear of regular things that are present in the world and can't be changed, such as illness, visiting the doctor, dying, and so on. Also for the timid and shy.

Emotional/Psychological Characteristics: Anxious; worried being around too many people and in small enclosed places; timid, shy, and nervous; fearful; nervous about speaking in front of people; afraid of the dark, of being by themselves, and of family members dying; fear of flying, high altitudes, and deep waters; nightmares.

Physical/General Indicators: Clammy hands; hyper-vigilant; frightened; sensitive to noise; hesitating and stuttering; shy; nervous; jittery; obsessive-compulsive.

Positive Outcome: Feels grounded and able to handle situations; relaxed and secure; has the courage to face fears.

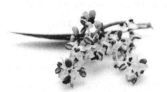

Olive (*Olea europaea*)

For mental and physical exhaustion from an extreme period of great struggle and anguish due to illness.

Emotional/Psychological Characteristics: Life has become too much to handle; drained with no energy or enthusiasm; inadequate diet; poor sleep; chronic worrying; lingering illness; extreme mental fatigue.

Physical/General Indicators: Very tired, needs rest, drained.

Positive Outcome: Renewed; feeling happier; strengthened and revitalized; more connected and with more sense to the body's needs.

~~~

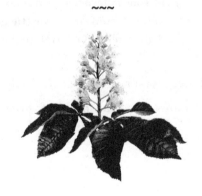

Red Chestnut (*Aesculus carnea*)

For those who are constantly anxious for the safety and well-being of other people, like friends and family.

Emotional/Psychological Characteristics: Too concerned over other people's problems and their lives; overly concerned with family members' health and safety.

Physical/General Indicators: Worry too much about other people's problems; over-protective of those they love; overly giving of oneself for others. Anxious; worried.

Positive Outcome: Able to care for others without being worried or over-controlling; nurturing to others without being neurotic; able to relax and feel secure.

~~~

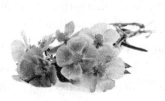

Rock Rose (Helianthemum nummularium)

For the feeling of shock, dread, and fear; nightmares.

Emotional/Psychological Characteristics: Anxious; nervous; panic attacks; terrified; traumatized from shock; brittle nerves; paralyzed with fear when natural disasters like earthquake and hurricanes occur.

Physical/General Indicators: Fearful, horrified, edgy; anxious.

Positive Outcome: More control in emergency situations; strong and secure; more grounded, less nervous.

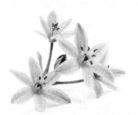

Star of Bethlehem (Ornithogalum umbellatum)

For those who suffered great distress due to a personal loss, accident, or a period of serious grief in their lives.

Emotional/Psychological Characteristics: Fragile; easily hurt physically and mentally; afraid; in a state of shock; disappointed; sad.

Physical/General Indicators: Distress; anguish; desolation; confused; incoherent speech. Self-induced mental conditions.

Positive Outcome: Handles situations in a calmer way; less scared and stronger inside; more in control; feeling calm and more whole.

~~~

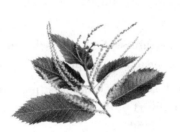

Sweet Chestnut (Castanea sativa)

For people who have reached the limit of their strength and have no energy reserve left.

Emotional/Psychological Characteristics: Hopelessness; desperation; mental torment; sadness and emptiness; feels rejected by God and lacks the ability to keep going; a total breakdown.

Physical/General Indicators: Drained; dejected and doomed; surrender.

Positive Outcome: Uplifted and restored; feels positive; more trusting spiritually; at ease, free, and liberated.

~~~

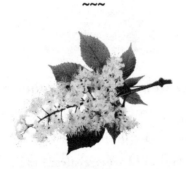

White Chestnut (Aesculus hippocastanum)

For people who experience constant unwanted, undesirable, or worrisome thoughts and cannot stop them; nervousness, tension, and insomnia.

Emotional/Psychological Characteristics: Mental state is one of continual brain chatter and swirling thoughts; unable to sleep; restless; unable to focus.

Physical/General Indicators: Tight muscles around the face and jaws; distress; tense; headaches, especially around the forehead.

Positive Outcome: A sense of quietness; peaceful and clear mind; focused and able to divert or discard the distressing thoughts when they try to enter the mind.

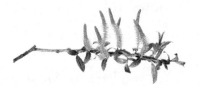

Willow (Salix vitellina)

For people who feel that life has treated them unjustly; who live life feeling angry, offended, and discouraged.

Emotional/Psychological Characteristics: Blame others for their failures; a negative life pattern; bitterness; gloomy; thinks that life is unfair.

Physical/General Indicators: Defensive; withdrawn; resentful; moody, pessimistic; negative.

Positive Outcome: Able to make positive changes; accept own mistakes; able to forgive others; optimistic; not as easily irritated.

Flower Remedy Self-Help Assessment

How to determine your custom remedy:

Read each statement and check all that apply. Go with your initial response; if you have to think about it, skip that statement. Don't limit your choices. After completing the assessment, circle the remedy names with two or more checks. Those are the remedies that will be helpful. Ideally, limit the number of remedies you use to six or fewer.

Agrimony

_____ I hide my feelings behind a façade of cheerfulness

_____ I dislike arguments and often give in to avoid conflict

_____ I turn to food, work, alcohol, drugs, etc. when down

Aspen

_____ I feel anxious without knowing why

_____ I have a secret fear that something bad will happen

_____ I wake up feeling anxious

Beech

_____ I get annoyed by the habits of others

_____ I focus on others' mistakes

_____ I am critical and intolerant

Centaury

_____ I often neglect my own needs to please

_____ I find it difficult to say "no"

_____ I tend to be easily influenced

Cerato

_____ I constantly second-guess myself

_____ I seek advice, mistrusting my own intuition

_____ I often change my mind out of confusion

Cherry Plum

_____ I'm afraid I might lose control of myself

_____ I have sudden fits of rage

_____ I feel like I'm going crazy

Chestnut Bud

_____ I make the same mistakes over and over

_____ I don't learn from my experience

_____ I keep repeating the same patterns

Chicory

_____ I need to be needed and want my loved ones close

_____ I feel unloved and unappreciated by my family

_____ I easily feel slighted and hurt

Clematis

_____ I often feel spacey and absent-minded

_____ I find myself unable to concentrate for long

_____ I get drowsy and sleep more than necessary

Crab Apple

_____ I am overly concerned with cleanliness

_____ I feel unclean or physically unattractive

_____ I tend to obsess over little things

Elm

_____ I feel overwhelmed by my responsibilities

_____ I don't cope well under pressure

_____ I have temporarily lost my self-confidence

Gentian

_____ I become discouraged with small setbacks

_____ I am easily disheartened when faced with difficulties

_____ I am often skeptical and pessimistic

Gorse

_____ I feel hopeless and can't see a way out

_____ I lack faith that things could get better in my life

_____ I feel sullen and depressed

Heather

_____ I am obsessed with my own troubles

_____ I dislike being alone and I like to talk

_____ I usually bring conversations back to myself

Holly

_____ I am suspicious of others

_____ I feel discontented and unhappy

_____ I am full of jealousy, mistrust, or hate

Honeysuckle

_____ I'm often homesick for the "way it was"

_____ I think more about the past than the present

_____ I often think about what might have been

Hornbeam

_____ I often feel too tired to face the day ahead

_____ I feel mentally exhausted

_____ I tend to put things off

Impatiens

_____ I find it hard to wait for things

_____ I am impatient and irritable

_____ I prefer to work alone

Larch

_____ I lack self-confidence

_____ I feel inferior and often become discouraged

_____ I never expect anything but failure

Mimulus

_____ I am afraid of things such as spiders, illness, etc.

_____ I am shy, overly sensitive, and modest

_____ I get nervous and embarrassed

Mustard

_____ I get depressed without any reason

_____ I feel my moods swinging back and forth

_____ I get gloomy feelings that come and go

Oak

_____ I tend to overwork and keep on in spite of exhaustion

_____ I have a strong sense of duty and never give up

_____ I neglect my own needs in order to complete a task

Olive

_____ I feel completely exhausted, physically and/or mentally
_____ I am totally drained of all energy with no reserves left
_____ I've just been through a long period of illness or stress

Pine

_____ I feel unworthy and inferior
_____ I often feel guilty
_____ I blame myself for everything that goes wrong

Red Chestnut

_____ I'm overly concerned and worried about my loved ones
_____ I'm distressed and disturbed by other people's problems
_____ I worry that harm may come to those I love

Rock Rose

_____ I sometimes feel terror and panic
_____ I become helpless and frozen when afraid
_____ I suffer from nightmares

Rock Water

_____ I set high standards for myself
_____ I am strict with my health, work and/or spiritual
discipline
_____ I am very self-disciplined, always striving for perfection

Scleranthus

_____ I find it difficult to make decisions
_____ I often change my opinions
_____ I have intense mood swings

Star of Bethlehem

_____ I feel devastated due to a recent shock

_____ I am withdrawn due to traumatic events in my life

_____ I have never recovered from loss or fright

Sweet Chestnut

_____ I feel extreme mental or emotional heartache

_____ I have reached the limits of my endurance

_____ I am in complete despair, all hope gone

Vervain

_____ I get high-strung and very intense

_____ I try to convince others of my way of thinking

_____ I am sensitive to injustice, almost fanatical

Vine

_____ I tend to take charge of projects, situations, etc.

_____ I consider myself a natural leader

_____ I am strong-willed, ambitious and often bossy

Walnut

_____ I'm experiencing change in life—a move, new job, etc.

_____ I get drained by people or situations

_____ I want to be free to follow my own ambitions

Water Violet

_____ I give the impression that I'm aloof

_____ I prefer to be alone when overwhelmed

_____ I often don't connect with people

White Chestnut

_____ I am constantly thinking unwanted thoughts

_____ I repeatedly relive unhappy events or arguments

_____ I'm unable to sleep at times because I can't stop thinking

Wild Oat

_____ I can't find my path in life

_____ I am drifting in life and lack direction

_____ I am ambitious but don't know what to do

Wild Rose

_____ I am apathetic and resigned to whatever happens

_____ I have the attitude, "It doesn't matter anyhow"

_____ I feel no joy in life

Willow

_____ I feel resentful and bitter

_____ I have difficulty forgiving and forgetting

_____ I think life is unfair and have a "Poor me" attitude

Source: Trinity School of Natural Health

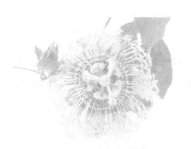

Appendix II

Herbs

Herbs have played an important role in our daily lives for centuries. Records dating back to 1500 BC tell us how people used herbs. I believe that in ancient times, people had an intuitive sense that healing comes from within, that herbs are a vital part of the healing process, and that the body possesses an innate ability to heal naturally without the need of unnatural substances, just the way God intended us to be. Herbs affect many processes in the human body; they correct and normalize imbalances, as well as cleanse, detoxify, and build the health of all the body systems. Herbs are remedies that can be ingested internally or applied externally.

Because herbs have a direct influence on the physical body, knowing what part of the body we want to assist and restore helps us select the appropriate herbs' action. Like minerals, herbs work in synergy; they need the support of each other, and this combined effort enhances the efficiency of their action. Also, like minerals, they sometimes play as a soloist, addressing issues by themselves.

One way herbs are categorized is by their specific actions on each of the body's systems and conditions, meaning how they work and the impact they have on the body. Though most plants have more than one action, the body innately knows and recognizes these actions and which system to heal.

Herbal actions correspond to each of the body systems; they stimulate, protect, soften, tone, relax, restore, soothe, and strengthen these systems. Sometimes a single action serves different purposes. For example, a nervine action relaxes the nerves, stimulates, and tones and nourishes the nervous system. Nervine action herbs have an affinity to the nervous system and are useful in managing nervousness, irritability, and anxiety.

Before we get into specific herbs, it's helpful for you to understand how herbs work. This list of herbal actions includes those that relate to anxiety:

Adaptogen. Herbs that help the body resist and deal with stress. They assist the adrenal glands, which are responsible for regulating stress in the body.

Alterative. Herbs that support and regenerate body functions and build strength and energy.

Anticatarrhal. Herbs that help expel excess mucus from the body, including the sinuses and lungs.

Anti-inflammatory. Herbs that help diminish inflammation or inflammatory issues in the body by assisting and stimulating the natural processes of the body.

Antimicrobial. Herbs that help strengthen the body's defensive mechanism against infectious organisms, destroying them and expelling illness.

Antispasmodic. Herbs that soothe muscle tension, muscle pain, and muscle spasms. Some antispasmodic herbs also help relax the smooth muscles of specific body systems and organs like the digestive system, the stomach, the intestines, and the bladder. They relieve emotional tension as well.

Astringent. Herbs that contain a chemical called tannins, which affix themselves to mucus membranes, the skin, and other body tissue to alleviate inflammation and irritation.

Bitter. The bitter taste of these herbs triggers the release of certain hormones that stimulate bile flow and digestive juices. These herbs aid poor digestion and improve absorption of nutrients; they also assist in gallbladder and liver detoxification.

Carminative. Plants with volatile oils that help digestive health by releasing gas and relieving inflammation and sharp pain.

Demulcent. Herbs that are soothing to the mucus membrane of the upper respiratory tract, the stomach, and tissues of the bowels, the bladder, and the lungs.

Diaphoretic. Herbs that promote perspiration, which helps the body get rid of toxins through the skin. They also stimulate circulation.

Diuretic. Herbs that have purgative properties. They help the body get rid of excess fluid; they promote the production and elimination of urine; they also help stimulate the kidneys, thereby helping flush away toxins and waste.

Emmenagogue. Herbs that tone and normalize the female reproductive system and stimulate menstrual flow.

Emollient. Herbs that restore moisture externally and internally. They have a mucilaginous effect. Used topically, they protect and soothe the skin. Used internally, they lubricate, moisten, and repair.

Expectorant. Herbs that stimulate even as they soothe and relax the bronchioles. They encourage the expelling of mucus from the lungs and loosen and thin mucus in the airway passages.

Hepatic: Herbs that tone and strengthen the liver; they may increase the flow of bile.

Hypotensive: Herbs that slow abnormally elevated blood pressure.

Laxative. Herbs that stimulate the bowels to empty and eliminate, usually used for constipation and in cleansing of the bowels.

Nervine. Herbs that support the nervous system. They are restorative and strengthening. They can be calming and relaxing, but also stimulating to the nerves.

Rubefacients: Herbs that provide cleansing and nourishment to the skin by increasing blow flow.

Tonic. Herbs that are tonifying and strengthening to the body's systems. They enhance general health by nurturing the whole body.

Vulnerary: Herbs that encourage skin wound healing; they also promote the healing of stomach ulcers.

Herbs known to aid in anxiety and stress

5-HTP (*Hydroxytryptophan*)

Appetite suppressant, anti-depressant

5-HTP is an amino acid produced by the body and it is a precursor to serotonin, a neurotransmitter responsible for regulating mood and anxiety. Low levels of serotonin affect sleep, appetite, and sexual behavior, this neurotransmitter increases the production of serotonin, therefore helping with anxiety, depression, weight gain, and sleep disorders like insomnia.

Caution: Do not take more than the recommended dosage. If taking prescription or over-the-counter medication, consult a health care practitioner before taking this supplement. Seek the advice of a health care practitioner if nursing or pregnant. Do not take with ADHD.

~~~

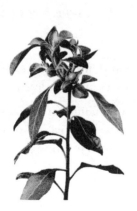

Ashwagandha *(Withania somnifera)*

Adaptogen, sedative, calmative, anti-stress

Ashwagandha works as a general tonic which is soothing to the nervous system. Ashwagandha is an adaptogenic herb that is restorative to the adrenal glands, therefore helping in regulating and resisting stress. It helps to lower cortisol levels, decreases anxiety and depression, and assists with insomnia. It supports thought clarity, thyroid health, the immune system, reproductive system, and the endocrine system.

Caution: If a thyroid condition exists, consult your healthcare provider before taking ashwagandha.

~~~

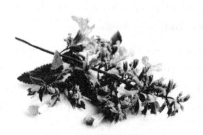

Catnip (*Nepeta cataria*)

Nervine, sedative

Soothing to the nervous system, promotes relaxation, calms anxiety, assists in sleep, nervousness, and restlessness.

Caution: Avoid during pregnancy and breastfeeding. Consult your doctor for use in children. May cause drowsiness and sleepiness. Avoid if scheduled for surgery. Can cause menstruation and may exacerbate heavy periods.

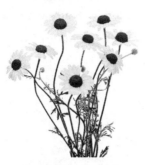

Chamomile *(Matricaria recutita)*

Calmative, nervine, digestive tonic, sedative

Relaxing to the nervous system and supporting to the adrenal glands and the parasympathetic nervous system. Helps anxiety, insomnia, irritability. Also helps in emotional sensitivity and nervousness, tension, and worry.

Caution: In rare cases, there have been reports of allergic reactions to chamomile. Chamomile may cause severe reactions in people allergic to ragweed, asters, and chrysanthemums.

~~~

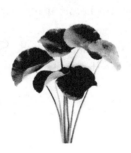

Gotu Kola *(Centella asiatica)*

Adaptogen, nervine, hypotensive

Supports the nervous system, helps with anxiety and depression, lowers stress, helps with insomnia. Gotu kola is a brain tonic that helps brain circulation, function, and concentration. It's also an adrenal gland tonic, helping with adrenal exhaustion.

Caution: Overdose may cause dizziness. Not recommended for long-term use.

~~~

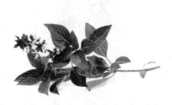

Holy Basil *(Ocimum tenuiflorum)*

Adaptogen, antidepressant, anti-anxiety

Not the common basil we know, holy basil is an adaptogen with energizing and invigorating properties. It relieves stress and anxiety; eases inflammation; is known for its tonifying effects to the body, mind and spirit; aids in sleep problems, memory, fatigue, and sexual issues.

Caution: Consult your doctor before using. May interact with medications. Do not use if you are pregnant, trying to become pregnant, or breastfeeding. May lower blood sugar, decrease fertility, and promote bleeding. Avoid it use if sensitive or allergic to plants in the mint family.

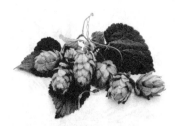

Hops *(Humulus lupulus)*

Nervine, sedative, tranquilizer

Supports the nerves, the central nervous system, helps sleep, muscle spasms, and relieves anxiety.

Caution: Not recommended for people suffering from depression.

~~~

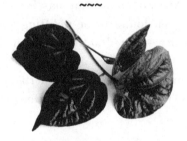

Kava kava *(Piper methysticum)*

Anxiolytic, relaxant, sedative

Good for anxiety disorders, depression, stress, nervousness, tension, and insomnia. Researchers say that kava kava may be one of the most effective herbs for anxiety and stress.

Caution: Do not use while driving a motor vehicle, when operating machinery or in conjunction with alcohol. Not to be taken for periods of time longer than three months. Do not take if you are under eighteen years of age, pregnant, or lactating. If you have liver problems, use alcohol frequently, or take any medication, consult a healthcare professional prior to use. Kava kava should only be used in small doses and for a short period of time. Never exceed the recommended dose and keep away from children.

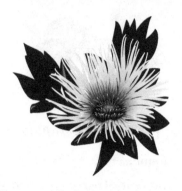

Kanna *(Sceletium tortuosum)*

Sedative, calmative, anti-depressant, relaxant

This is a South African plant that has been used for centuries for stress. It has been found to be uplifting and sedative, relieve stress and the anxiety-related activities in the amygdala (brain's emotional center), help sleep and depressive feelings and thoughts. When taken in combination with other herbs, vitamins, and minerals as well as L-Theanine, it works well for managing anxiety or panic attacks.

~~~

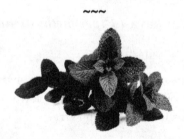

Lemon Balm *(Melissa Officinalis)*

Anti-depressive, nervine

Helps ease anxiety, tension, depression, and heart palpitations. Good for insomnia and soothes the nervous system.

Caution: Not for long-term use. Avoid use if pregnant or breast-feeding, or if a thyroid condition exists. May lower blood sugar in people with diabetes and hypoglycemia. Avoid if scheduled for surgery. Do not take with sleep aid medications. Consult your doctor prior to use.

~~~

L-Theanine

Anxiolytic

This is a non-essential amino acid that is found in green and black tea. It encourages relaxation without sedative effects and enhances concentration. Though it is not an herb, it's listed here for its support during times of stress and anxiety. L-Theanine may be more effective when combined with other herbs that relieve anxiety and stress than on its own.

~~~

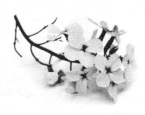

Motherwort (*Leonurus cardiaca*)

Nervine, hypotensive, sedative

This herb is a heart tonic; it calms, assists in anxiety, tension, and fear that may be due to hormonal changes related to menopause, and heart palpitations caused by stress and anxiety.

Caution: Avoid if pregnant or breastfeeding. May cause drowsiness or sleepiness. Consult with your doctor before using if taking a sleep aid medication.

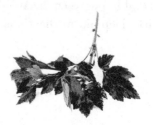

Mugwort: *(Artemisia vulgaris)*

Nervine, antidepressant

Mugwort's nervine effects help with anxiety, restlessness, insomnia, irritability, fatigue and depression.

Caution: Not recommended during pregnancy and breastfeeding.

~~~

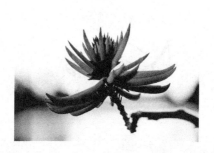

Mulungu Bark (*Erythrina mulungu*)

Sedative, hypotensive, nervine

Sooths the nervous system. Sedative effects promote deep healthy sleep patterns. Helpful with anxiety, fear, stress, depression, mania, shock, and distress. Relieves muscle pain.

Caution: If you are taking blood pressure medication, consult with your doctor before taking mulungu. Avoid if you have low blood pressure. May cause drowsiness. Do not use while driving a motor vehicle or operating machinery. Do not use in conjunction with alcohol.

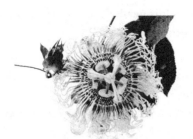

Passion Flower: *(Passiflora)*

Anxiolytic, calmative, nervine, sedative

Supports the central nervous system and the parasympathetic nervous system. Stress relieving and calming to the nerves. Has been used for sleep disorders and insomnia for centuries. It produces deep relaxation and calms an over-thinking mind, especially when a person can't fall asleep because the mind can't shut down. It helps decrease anxiety, hysteria, nervousness; aids in depression; helps with heart weakness and heart palpitations; helps with hyperactivity disorders; lowers blood pressure, and prevents tachycardia.

Caution: May cause drowsiness. Do not use while driving a motor vehicles or operating heavy machinery.

~~~

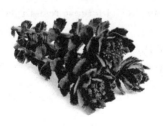

Rhodiola *(Rosea)*

Adaptogen

Helps the body adapt to stress. Energizing, aids with anxiety, stress, and mental exhaustion. Decreases mental fatigue and depressive moods. Assists in regulating of heartbeat. Improves memory.

Although more research is needed, it may stimulate dopamine, nor-epinephrine and serotonin activity.

Caution: Check with your doctor before using. May cause drowsiness. Avoid if pregnant, breastfeeding, or are taking prescription medications. Not for long-term use. Not recommended in autoimmune conditions. May lower blood sugar and blood pressure.

~~~

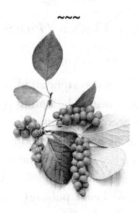

Schisandra (*Schisandra chinensis*)

Adaptogen

Combined with energizing herbs like ginseng and B vitamins, it makes a powerful formula to increase resistance to stress and relieve anxiety. It helps increase stamina and enhances endurance, and is therefore helpful to the adrenal glands and adrenal exhaustion, heart palpitations, and the nervous system.

Caution: Do not take while pregnant or breastfeeding. Do not take if epileptic.

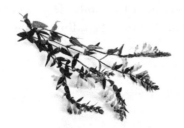

Skullcap (*Scutellaria lateriflora*)

Sedative, nervine, relaxant

Calming to the nervous system, helping stress and anxiety, nervousness, nervous tension, hysteria, insomnia, muscular twitching, irritability, and circulating thoughts.

Caution: Do not take while pregnant or breastfeeding, or if scheduled for surgery.

~~~

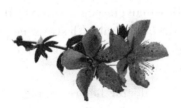

St. John's Wort *(Hypericum perforatum)*

Nervine, anti-depressant, hypotensive, relaxant, sedative, serotonergic

Known for relieving anxiety, depression, and tension, it eases excessive fear, irritability due to hormonal changes in menopause. Helps with insomnia and nightmares.

Caution: Large doses may cause severe reactions to sun exposure. St. John's Wort is known to interact with many prescription medications, so consult your healthcare provider before taking it. It is unsafe for pregnant or breastfeeding mothers or for women planning to conceive. Always consult with your doctor before taking

St. John's Wort or giving it to a child. If you are taking St. John's Wort, tell your doctor before scheduling surgery.

~~~

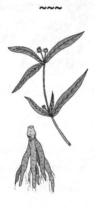

Suma *(Hebanthe eriantha)*

Adaptogen

Sometimes called Brazilian ginseng because of its energizing effects to the body. Helps the body deal with stress; helps balance the adrenal glands and high cortisol levels; helps balance hormones; aids in sexual issues and memory.

Caution: Consult your doctor before taking. Lowers blood sugar. Avoid during pregnancy or breastfeeding.

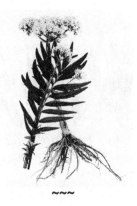

~~~

Valerian Root: *(Valeriana officinalis)*

Nervine, sedative, hypotensive

Supports the adrenal glands and the nervous system, eases muscle tension, has tranquilizing effects, is a muscle relaxer, and mild pain reliever. It's a relaxing herb for hypertension when stress is the cause. It assists in nervousness, anxiety, and insomnia. Promotes deep sleep.

Caution: Consult your doctor before use. May cause drowsiness. Do not use while driving a motor vehicle or operating machinery. Do not use in conjunction with alcohol. Avoid use if pregnant, breast-feeding, or scheduled for surgery.

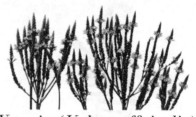

Vervain *(Verbena officinalis)*

Nervine, sedative, hypotensive

A relaxant that helps ease stress and tension; helps anxiety, nervous exhaustion, and tics; strengthens the nervous system; supports the immune system and the parasympathetic nervous system. It relieves depression and feelings of sadness and gloom.

Caution: Avoid use if pregnant.

~~~

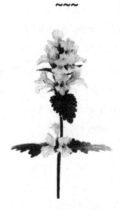

Wood betony: *(Stachys officinalis)*

Hypotensive, antianxiety, nervine, sedative, relaxant

Helps us reconnect in body and mind, and deal with negative emotions. It also aids the digestive system, supports the nervous system and the pineal gland, helps with nervous exhaustion and tension, helps relieve anxiety, hyperactivity, restlessness, and depression.

Caution: Not recommended for use during pregnancy or while breastfeeding. Stop use if scheduled for surgery. Consult with your doctor before taking because there is evidence of interaction with blood pressure medication.

Herbal combinations

Like essential oils, flower essences, and minerals, herbs work very well in combination for many different types of ailments, but especially for stress and anxiety. These are some combination of herbs known to support our body in times of stress and anxiety.

Adaptogenic or restorative herbs

These herbs restore and bring balance to glands and organs. They help the body cope, adapt and resist high levels of stress, as well as assist the body in fighting negative and toxic stress and to alleviate stress.

Some of these herbs are ashwagandha, amla, bacopa, cordyceps, dang shen, dong quai, eleuthero, ginseng, gotu kola, holy basil, hyssop, jiaogulan, licorice root, maca, maitake, milk thistle, rhodiola, schisandra, and suma. Most of these herbs also strengthen the immune system, because high levels of stress can weaken and depress the immune system; they also prevent and decrease fatigue and alleviate depression.

Look for herbal combinations that help specific symptoms. For example, herbs for stress that will support the nervous system include chamomile, catnip, hops, gotu kola, lemon balm, lavender, sceletium tortuosum, skullcap, and valerian root.

Herbs that tonify the adrenal glands include ashwagandha, astragalus, cordyceps, eleuthero root, ginseng, gotu kola, gynostemma penthaphyllum, lycium barbarum, schisandra chinensis, rhadiola, and suma.

Herbs that help relax the body and mind, aid with insomnia, and support restful sleep include chamomile, gaba, gotu kola, hops, kava kava, lavender, lemon balm, passionflower, skullcap, and valerian root.

Nervine herbs

Nervine herbs support the nervous system; they have calming and uplifting effects, reduce tension and fatigue, ease mental stress, relieve racing thoughts, reduce nervousness, stress, worry, and restlessness. Some of these herbs are catnip, chamomile, hops, lavender, lemon balm, skullcap, passionflower, oat tops, skullcap, valerian root, and wood betony.

Calmative or relaxant herbs

These herbs calm and relax the nervous system, reduce nervous tension, nervous stomachs, and insomnia.

Some of these herbs are chamomile, catnip, bacopa, hops, kava kava, lavender, lemon balm, mugwort, motherwort, sceletium tortuosum, skullcap, passionflower, and valerian.

Sedative herbs

Sedative herbs are calming and produce a tranquilizing effect. They soothe and induce sleep. They include chamomile, hops, gaba, gotu kola, kava kava, lavender, lemon balm, mulungu bark, passionflower, skullcap, and valerian root, and wood betony.

Chinese herbal formulas

Chinese medicine has a vast number of herbs for stress, anxiety, the immune system, and nervous system, for strengthening the adrenal glands, and for balancing and energizing all five constitutional types, which are also called the five elements (fire, wood, earth, metal, and water). Some of those

herbs are Asian ginseng root, astragalus, cordyceps, eleuthero root, gynostemma, hoelen, lycium barbarum, sclerotium.
penthaphyllum, polygala, and schisandra chinensis.

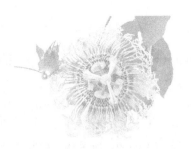

Appendix III

Essential Oils

Essential oils date back to ancient times when they were more valuable than gold. They were used for an array of purposes, including anointing, purification, embalming, and medicinal purposes. The two most well-known essential oils were frankincense and myrrh. Essential oils are mentioned frequently in the Bible.

Essential oils can help emotional balancing, soothe the nervous system, and ease stress and anxiety. Essential oils balance these emotions by reaching deep inside the amygdala, which is the center of the brain that processes emotions, to target emotions that are stuck and release them. The amygdala is part of the limbic system, which is located underneath the cerebrum on both sides of the thalamus. It's composed of a set of structures in our brain that handles emotions and memory. The parts that make up the limbic system are the amygdala, hippocampus, thalamus, hypothalamus, basal ganglia, and circulate gyrus.

The thalamus is concerned with things we hear, touch, and taste; it's the part of the brain that relays these emotions. When stimulated, the amygdala can create feelings of fear, anxiety, anger, and violence. If the amygdala is damaged, it can produce feelings of mellowing and no fear results. The hippocampus role is in forming new memory; it helps transform short-term memory into long-term memory. The hypothalamus regulates the autonomic nervous system, which is the mechanism in control of the "fight or flight" response. The hypothalamus also controls the endocrine system by activating the release of hormones (epinephrine and norepinephrine) into the bloodstream. It's the gland that controls hunger, sex, sleep, circadian rhythms, thirst, body temperature, and fatigue.

Limbic system

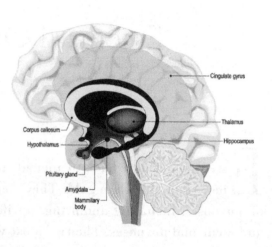

Essential oils helpful in managing anxiety

Essential oils may be used aromatically or topically; they may also be used in diffusers, massage, compresses, baths, scrubs, lotions, and sprays. Essential oils should be diluted with a carrier oil or massage oil before applying topically. Some essential oils can be very photosensitizing, and you should avoid applying them to skin that will be exposed to direct sunlight or ultraviolet light. Keep essential oils out of the reach of children. Consult your doctor before apply essential oils to children.

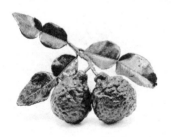

Bergamot *(Citrus bergamia)*

Calmative, antidepressant, relaxant

Origin: Ivory Coast, Italy

Its fresh essence calms and uplifts, helps relieve stress, and anxiety. Bergamot is also known to help with insomnia, compulsive/obsessive behaviors, fear, nervous indigestion, tension, muscle spasms, and moods.

Caution: Consult your doctor if you are pregnant, breastfeeding, or before using on children. Bergamot is a photosensitizing essential oil and should not be applied to skin that will be exposed to direct sunlight or ultraviolet light.

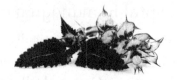

Clary Sage (*Salvia sclarea*)

Relaxant, calmative, antidepressant

Origin: France, USA

Used for a variety of applications, including depression, insomnia, nightmares, panic, stress, anxiety, tension, nervousness, and irritability. It balances and lifts mood, especially during the menstrual cycle and menopause.

~~~

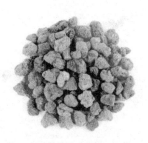

Frankincense (*Boswellia Carteri, sacra*)

Antidepressant, calmative, relaxant

Origin: Somalia

In ancient times, frankincense was valued more than gold. Its essence is woody and earthy. Researchers have found that frankincense chemically has a high concentration in sesquiterpenes, which aids in stimulating the limbic system of the brain, the emotional center, which is responsible for the feeling and the expression of emotions, the hypothalamus, pineal and pituitary glands. It's uplifting, stimulating, calming to the mind, soothes the spirit, promotes focus, relieves depression, relaxes muscles, helps in concentration, and eases anxiety, fear, nightmares, negativity, and stress.

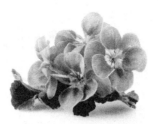

Geranium *(Pelargonium graveolens)*

Calmative, relaxant, nervine

Origin: Egypt, India

Geranium is stimulating; it may help tension, anxiety, stress, hyper-activity and insomnia, nervousness, depression, and nightmares. It also aids in the release of negativity such as negative memories.

~~~

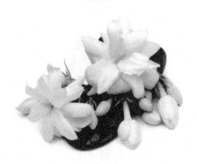

Jasmine *(Jasminum officinale)*

Antidepressant, calmative

Origin: India, Middle East, Asia

Jasmine is uplifting; it helps ease anxiety, stress, insomnia, depression, nightmares, and is soothing to the nervous system.

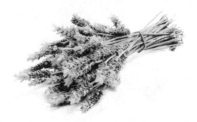

Lavender *(Lavandula angustifolia)*

Sedative, relaxant

Origin: France, USA

Relaxing and comforting, lavender calms the nerves, supports sleep, and helps with insomnia. It may help depression, anxiety, emotions, and tension.

~~~

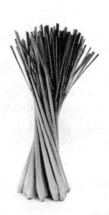

Lemongrass: *(Cymbopogon flexuosus)*

Sedative, relaxant

Origin: Guatemala, India, Sri Lanka, Burma, Thailand

The exquisite fresh, earthy, citrusy fragrance of lemongrass is known to many for its numerous uses and benefits. It is purifying and relaxing, reduces stress, and relaxes muscle tension.

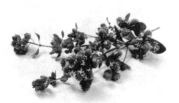

Marjoram *(Origanum majorana)*

Calmative, relaxant, nervine

Origin: Mediterranean, North Africa, Western Asia

Supporting to the parasympathetic nervous system, marjoram promotes calmness to anxiety, is soothing to nervous tension and nervousness, eases tensed muscles, and helps with insomnia and worry.

~~~

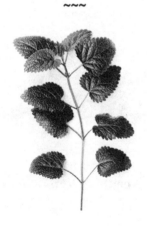

Melissa *(Melissa officinalis)*

Calmative, sedative, hypotensive

Origin: France, USA.

May help with anxiety, emotions of the heart, nervous conditions, depression, heart palpitations, nervousness, and insomnia. Its essence is invigorating, calming, and elevating, and it may also help in stabilizing emotions by unblocking the negative predicament a person may find himself in, restoring it to a positive disposition.

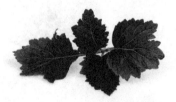

Patchouli *(Pogostemon cablin)*

Calmative, nervine, sedative

Origin: Name originated from South India, native to Southeast Asia

Its essence is tranquilizing, relaxing, and soothing. It tones the nerves, easing anxiety and relieving depression. It's uplifting, helping nervous fatigue and overthinking, as well as releasing deep unresolved emotions.

~~~

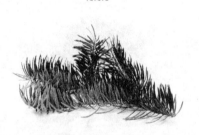

Pine Needle *(Pinus sylvestris)*

Stimulate, revitalize

Origin: Australia, Canada, Russia.

Invigorating and uplifting, pine needle eases tensed muscles and stress. It's rejuvenating for those with mental fatigue and adrenal glands exhaustion, nervous fatigue, nervousness, and depression. It helps increase blood pressure. It improves feelings of disillusionment, guilt, and self-deprecation.

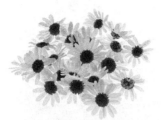

Roman Chamomile *(Chamomile nobile)*

Sedative, calmative

Origin: Italy, Hungary, Argentina, France, Belgium, UK, USA.

Eases stress and anxiety, depression, tension and muscle tension, nervous indigestion and nervousness, insomnia, PMS symptoms, and hyperactivity. Relieves negative feelings and negative thoughts. Supports the adrenal glands.

~~~

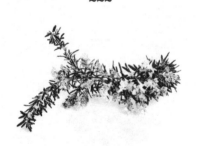

Rosemary (Salvia rosmarinus)

Antispasmodic, calmative, relaxant

Origin: Mediterranean

Rosemary brings peace, eases nervousness and tension, and promotes relaxation and meditation. With its marked effects on the brain and central nervous system, it clears the mind, improves focus, alertness, memory, and mood. It helps the weary, eases resentment, and relieves nightmares.

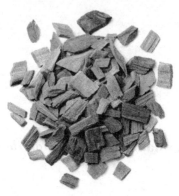

Sandalwood *(Santalum album)*

Calmative, sedative

Origin: India, Indonesia.

Sandalwood is energizing, assists in meditation, and promotes deep sleep. It has been used for depression, nervousness, nightmares, worry, and muscle tension.

~~~

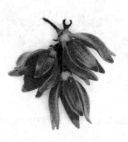

Ylang Ylang *(Cananga odorata)*

Nervine, antidepressant, sedative

Origin: Indonesia, Philippines.

Its fragrant and beautiful essence calms and relaxes. It eases anxiety, fear, shock, stress, nervousness, mental exhaustion, depression, tension, and fatigue. It's harmonizing, calms the heart, and helps palpitations, tachycardia, and hyperventilation. It supports in balancing blood pressure and assists in regulating heartbeat and insomnia.

Caution: For external use only. Avoid use during pregnancy or nursing, near eyes or mucous membranes. Consult your doctor before use if taking medications or using for children. Discontinue use and consult your doctor if any adverse reactions occur. Do not use directly on the skin; dilute with a carrier oil before applying topically. Do not apply to broken or irritated skin; if skin sensitivity occurs, discontinue use. Avoid sun exposure after topical use.

Essential oil blends

Essential oils work great singly but become powerful infusions when blended. Essential oil blends can address issues in a more complex way. Because blended oils complement one another, their specific medicinal properties have a stronger impact. A blend can create beautiful aromas. A custom blend can also create a special scent that, when needed by an individual, can be therapeutic, invigorating, and healing.

Below is a list of essential oil blends for specific purposes:

Allergy: Clove, eucalyptus, lavender, lemongrass, lemon, peppermint, tea tree.

Anxiety: Bergamot, frankincense, lavender, orange, rose and ylang ylang.

Breath: Eucalyptus, ginger, lavender, peppermint, pine needle, rosemary.

Calming blend: Bergamot, chamomile, cinnamon leaf, lavender, lemon, mandarin, pink grapefruit, orange, rose, ylang ylang.

Energy: Lemon, ginger, grapefruit, peppermint, frankincense, orange.

Focus: Basil, cinnamon leaf, frankincense, lavender, lemon, pine needle, rosemary.

Immunity: Clove bud, cinnamon bark, cinnamon leaf, citrus lemon, oregano, rosemary, thyme.

Sleep: Bergamot, frankincense, lavender, orange, sweet marjoram, sandalwood, ylang ylang.

Wellness: Cinnamon bark, ginger, lemon, orange, peppermint, pink grapefruit, spearmint.

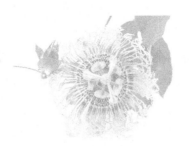

Appendix IV

Anxiety Source Worksheet

U se the following worksheet to help you identify the source(s) of your anxiety.

Your answers to these questions will help you identify the source(s) of your anxiety. Once you know the source(s), you can develop a plan to manage your issues and relieve your anxiety.

How stressed do you feel? Using a scale of 1-10, with 1 being the lowest and 10 being the highest, rank your stress level.

_____

Do you feel like you have too much going on?

_____

Are you attempting to multitask and feeling ineffective? Are you not coping well with the demands on your time?

_____

Do you feel overwhelmed and exhausted? Are you trying to handle too many things (home, family, work, etc.) at the same time?

_____

Are you concerned about your financial situation?

_____

If you are in a relationship, is it stable and solid or is it unstable and causing problems?

_____

Do you feel like you are emotionally stable? Or are there issues from your past or in your present such as hurt, anguish, anger, frustration, grudges, resentment, and bitterness that you think about regularly that cause pain?

_____

Are you grieving a loss of a person or situation?

_____

Have you experienced any recent major life changes? If so, what are they and how do you feel about them?

_____

Are you generally happy with your life overall, including family, relationships, general environment? If not, what areas are you not happy with?

_____

Do you feel like you are in control of your life or is something or someone else controlling you?

_____

Are you sleeping well?

_____

Is your diet balanced and healthful?

_____

Do you exercise regularly?

_____

Are you able to forgive people who have hurt you or do you hold grudges and fantasize about revenge?

_____

Are you alone? Or do you feel alone or isolated even when you are with others?

_____

Are you achieving your goals?

_____

Are your hormones balanced?

_____

Do you feel connected within yourself—mind, body, spirit?

_____

Are you grounded by and connected with the Holy Spirit?

_____

Review your answers to identify and prioritize the areas you need to work on. Some might be simple and quick to address; others will take more time and effort. As you make progress, update your answers on the worksheet.

To download a copy of this worksheet, visit
HealingBodiesandMinds.com.

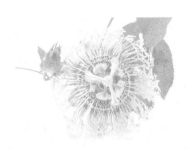

Glossary

Adaptogen: Herbs that help the body deal with stress, they help the body resist stress, and they support the adrenal glands since they are responsible for regulating stress in our body.

Adrenal glands: Small glands that are part of the endocrine system, located on the top of the kidneys, which produce hormones like adrenaline, and the steroids hormone aldosterone and cortisol.

Adrenalcorticotropic hormone: A hormone secreted by the pituitary gland that stimulates the adrenal glands to work properly and react to stress.

Adrenaline: A hormone produced by the adrenal glands that prepares the body for fight or flight response to fear, sensed threat, and panic. In stressful situations, it prepares the muscles for action and energy, increases heartbeat, strengthens the power of the heart contractions, increases breathing and carbohydrate metabolism.

Ailment: A minor illness.

Aldosterone: A hormone produced by the adrenal glands in the zona glomerulosa of the adrenal cortex. It is the primary mineralocorticoid hormone vital for sodium conservation in the kidneys, salivary glands, sweat glands, and the colon. It also signals the kidneys and the colon for the increase in the amount of sodium the body releases into the bloodstream or the amount of potassium released in the urine.

Anxiety attack: An apprehensive uneasiness or nervousness usually over an impending or anticipated ill; a state of being anxious.

Burnout: The feeling of being emotionally, physically, and mentally exhausted, usually from extreme and extended stress.

Cardiovascular: Relating to the heart and the blood vessels.

Chi: Also known as qi. Identified in Chinese medicine as the "vital force." The traditional Chinese viewpoint or philosophy believe that chi is the force that creates things and fixes them together.

Compress: A piece of cloth that has been soaked with an herbal infusion or extract to be applied to the affected skin area for wound healing and injuries.

Cope, coping skills: The ability to confront and deal with a job or responsibility, struggles, or difficulties calmly and successfully.

Cortisol: A hormone vital for general health, produced in the adrenal cortex, which is the outer part of the adrenal glands. It helps assist with memory formulation, helps control blood pressure and blood sugar levels, regulates metabolism, and helps reduce inflammation.

Deprecation: Self-depreciation, self-criticism.

Deprivation: A lack or denial of something considered a need.

Disease: A disorder of structure or function in a human, animal, or plant that impairs normal functioning, typically manifested by distinguishing signs and symptoms, and is not simply a direct result of a physical injury.

Disillusionment: Feeling of disappointment, discouragement.

Diuretic: An herbal property that helps the body excrete water when there is water retention.

Dopamine: A neurotransmitter and precursor of other substances including epinephrine.

Epidemic: A rapid spread of an infectious disease to a large number of people within a short period of time.

Epinephrine: A hormone mostly secreted by the medulla of the adrenal glands, also called adrenaline. Its primary functions are to increase cardiac output and increase glucose levels in the bloodstream.

Gonad: An organ that produces gametes; a testis or ovary.

Heart palpitations: A feeling of the heart fluttering, racing, skipping a beat, or pounding.

Herb: An aromatic plant with leaves, flowers, seeds, stems, and roots used in medicine, seasoning, or perfume.

Herbal action: The effect produced by an herb property.

Herbal infusion: The process of soaking herbs in water, allowing the water to absorb the flavor and properties before it's consumed.

Hypotensive: Low blood pressure.

Hypothalamus: A portion of the brain the size of an almond that contains several small nuclei with a variety of functions. Primarily the hypothalamus links the nervous system to the endocrine system via the pituitary gland.

Immune system: A group of cells, organs, and tissues that collectively operate to defend the body from diseases produced mainly by pathogens, bacteria, fungi, parasites, and viruses.

Lymphatic: The system consisting of a network of tissues and organs that help rid the body of toxins, waste, and other unwanted materials.

Nervine: An herbal property used to calm the nerves.

Nervous system: A network of nerve cells and fibers that conducts nerve impulses between parts of the body.

Night terror: Waking up from deep sleep feeling extreme fear and horror.

Nightmare: A frightening, terrifying, or unpleasant dream.

Obsessive-compulsive: The instinct or drive of a person to have to act repetitively to ease constant fears and emerging thoughts.

Palpitations: A rapid, strong, or irregular heartbeat.

Panic attack: An abrupt event of extreme fear or anxiety and physical symptoms, built on thoughts of threat rather than actual imminent danger.

Parasympathetic nervous system: Produces nearly the exact opposite effect as the sympathetic nervous system; it relaxes the body and slows down many elevated energy functions.

Phobia: A persistent and extreme fear of an object or situation.

Photosensitizing: A reaction caused by a chemical change from one molecule to another when exposed to sunlight, causing irritation, swelling, and dermatitis.

Pineal gland: An endocrine gland shaped like a pinecone located in the epithalamus, near the center of the brain between the two hemispheres, tucked in a groove where the two halves of the thalamus join. It produces melatonin, a serotonin-derived hormone that controls sleep patterns in both circadian and seasonal cycles.

Pituitary gland: About the size of a pea, the pituitary gland is a protrusion off the bottom of the hypothalamus at the base of the brain. It is crucial in controlling growth and development, as well as in the functioning of the other endocrine glands.

Qi: The life force in Chinese philosophy and medicine. See *Chi.*

Quivering: Shaking or trembling with a slight, rapid motion.

Restorative: Having the ability to restore health and strength.

Serotonin: A compound found in blood platelets and in the serum, which constricts blood vessels and also performs as a neurotransmitter.

Serum lipids: A profile that measures cardiovascular risk predictions. The test includes four basic parameters: total cholesterol, LDL cholesterol, HDL cholesterol, and triglycerides.

Sleep disturbance: Sleep disruption that involves the quality, the time, and the right amount of sleep needed.

Stimulant: A substance that increases levels of physiological or nervous activity in the body.

Stress: A state of mental or emotional strain and tension resulting from unpleasant or very challenging situations.

Sympathetic nervous system: Excite the body's fight or flight, as well as continually being active to maintain the body's homeostasis homeodynamics.

Synchronize: To cause something to occur at the same time or rate.

Tachycardia: A rapid heartbeat that is out of proportion to age and level of exertion or activity.

Thymus gland: A lymphoid organ located in the upper anterior part of the chest, right behind the sternum, between the lungs. It produces T cells for the immune system. This gland becomes much smaller in size at the approach of puberty.

Vibration: A fluctuation of the part of a fluid or an electro-magnetic wave.

Vibrational infusion: The frequency vibration that flowers emit into a fluid or water

Visualization: It is to see or create a picture of a place or something in our minds.

Vitamin: Any of a group of organic compounds essential for normal growth and nutrition.

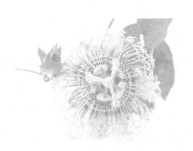

Resources

Anxiety and Depression Association of America (ADAA) (adaa.org)

Bernard Jensen, Ph. D. *The Chemistry of Man*. Indiana: Whitman Publications 2007.

Brenton G. Yorkgason, Ph.D. PDR *People's Desk Reference for Essential Oils*. USA: Essential Science 1999

Brilliant Body Series: Julie A. DeVisser, *Glandular System*; Joanne Mied and Steven Horne, *Nervous System*; Hannah Pavick, *Immune System*. Nature's Sunshine.

David Hoffmann, FNIMH, AHG. *Herbs for Healthy Aging*. Vermont: Healing Arts Press 2007

Everyday Health (everydayhealth.com)

Healthline.com

James Green, Herbalist. *The Male Herbal*. USA: Crossing Press 1991, 2007

James L. Wilson and Jonathan V Wright. *Adrenal Fatigue: The 21st Century Stress Syndrome*. California: Smart Publications 2001

Mark Pedersen ND, *Nutritional Herbology*. Indiana: Whitman Publications 2010

Mastering Mood and Emotions an Herbal and Nutritional support class seminar (Nature's Sunshine) Utah: 2018

Mechthild Scheffer. *The Encyclopedia of Bach Flower Therapy*. Vermont: Healing Arts Press 1999

Medical News Today (medicalnewstoday.com)

MedicineNet.com

Phil James, *God's Little Instruction Book for Women*. Oklahoma: Honors Books

Steven H. Horne, *The ABC Herbal: A Simplified Guide to Natural Health Care for Children*. Indiana: Whitman Publications 1992, 2005, 2007

Steven Horne and Kimberly Balas, *The Comprehensive Guide to Nature's Sunshine Products 6th Edition*. Utah: Tree of Life Publications 2003, 2009, 2012, 2014

Taking Charge of your Health & Wellbeing, University of Minnesota, takingcharge.csh.umn.edu

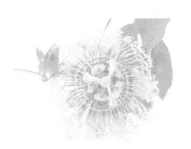

Acknowledgments

First and foremost, I want to thank God for His goodness and His mercies that are new every morning, for without Him this book would never have been written.

To my husband Frank: Thank you for your unwavering support and love, for taking care of me in my most difficult moments.

I have been blessed with the most beautiful family and I want to thank all of them. They are the reason I keep going. They fill my life with such joy and happiness. They share an enormous unconditional love for one another, supporting and protecting each other no matter the circumstances or situation.

To my sons Bryant and Kenneth: You are the best children any parent could ever ask for. You have always been there for me, you have always listened, and you always do what's right. Thank you for growing up to be such wonderful men.

To my niece, Greeny Marquez: You're not only a niece, you're my best friend, always supporting everything I do and being there for me.

To my sisters Agueda and Monica: Thank you for guiding me spiritually and emotionally through that difficult stage in my life.

I'm fortunate to be surrounded by good friends—friends who are also professionals who helped me with advice and support when I was in the middle of my anxiety crisis, who were there as I healed, and who continue to be with me today. I was never alone. I want to express my deepest gratitude to Dr. Ira Shafran, MD, Dr. Vraj Panara, MD., Sue Clemons CNHP, RN, MH, Dr. Rick Clemons ND, MH, and Dr. Rex W. Roffler, DC.

A special thank you goes to Kathy Van Dingstee, Kenneth Nunez, and Monica Nunez for reading the manuscript before it was published.

Finally, I want to thank Jacquelyn Lynn and Jerry Clement for all their great work and professionalism in bringing this project to fruition. Jacquelyn has always been helpful, kind, patient, and very thorough. She has been involved in all the aspects, making me feel like it's her own work.

Dominga Nunez

About Dominga Nunez, ND, CNHP

Natural medicine enhances and completes Dominga's life. It is one of her greatest joys to have the opportunity of helping people in a holistic way, and to make a positive impact in their lives.

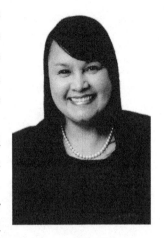

Dominga's interest in natural medicine started when she was a child in the Dominican Republic. She would see her mother make her own herbal infusions, poultices, and tinctures. Her mother did this to help Dominga and her siblings heal, for better health, and to cleanse their bodies. When she grew up, Dominga did the same thing for herself and her children. Her interest in natural health was recharged and reinforced throughout her life because she spent all her career time working in the natural health field.

Dominga Nunez is a Holistic Health Practitioner with a passion for natural health. She graduated from the University of Natural Medicine with a bachelor's degree in Natural Health Sciences and from Trinity School of Natural Health as a Certified Natural Health Professional (CNHP) and as a Naturopathic Doctor. She is board certified as a Holistic Health Practitioner with the American Association for Drugless Practitioners.

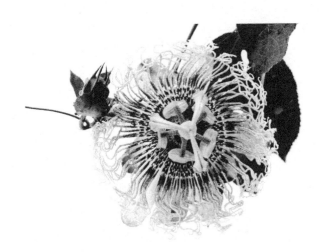

Download a free copy of the

Anxiety Source
Worksheet

Visit
HealingBodiesandMinds.com

Made in the USA
Las Vegas, NV
12 May 2024